SPECIAL FEATURES

SPECIAL FEATURES

Techniques for One-of-a-Kind Beauty from J. Roy Helland

BY J. ROY HELLAND
AND MEG F. SCHNEIDER
Illustrations by Jack Eckstein
Created by The Miller Press, Inc.

M. Evans and Company, Inc.
New York

Library of Congress Cataloging in Publication Data

Helland, J. Roy.
  Special features.

  1. Beauty, Personal. 2. Cosmetics.   I. Schneider,
Meg F.   II. Title.
RA778.H448   1985   646.7'26   84-21262

ISBN 0-87131-442-8

M. Evans and Company, Inc.
216 East 49 Street
New York, New York 10017

Design by James L. McGuire

Manufactured in the United States of America

9 8 7 6 5 4 3 2 1

To all the ladies, gentlemen, and "really women" who have so kindly lent their faces, hair, and time for my experimentation.

Roy Helland

To Marilyn,

Thanks for giving me a start, and always being there to help me continue. That's family for you . . .

Meg F. Schneider

My thanks to Bob Kelly, who for years has shared his knowledge, experience, and products with me, and to Meg, who has put my thoughts into words and sentences.
R.H.

I would like to acknowledge Maureen Heffernan for her creative editorial eye, and everyone else at M. Evans for their boundless enthusiasm.
M.F.S.

Contents

About the Authors

J. Roy Helland has blended his love of theater with his natural talents for hair and makeup into a successful twenty-three-year career.

Roy's interest in the art of character makeup was kindled while he was studying drama in school. He enthusiastically went on to master those techniques while pursuing a performing career. As time passed Roy realized that his true interests and talents lay in creating the exterior image of a character rather than in dancing or acting the part; and so he opened a beauty salon in Los Angeles.

After six years of building his own business, Roy moved to New York where he began working at Kenneth's, and soon struck out on his own where his experience in live theater and the "real life" arenas paid off.

Roy works primarily in theater and film. His theater work includes *Three Penny Opera, Streamers, Pirates of Penzance, The Real Thing*, and Mikhail Baryshnikov's production of *Cinderella*. His film credits number *A Bridge Too Far, Sophie's Choice*, and *Silkwood* among them. He is the favored artist of Linda Ronstadt, Meryl Streep, Liv Ullmann, and Mariel Hemingway, among others.

Roy believes the single most important talent he possesses is his ability to see the potential of the whole, and at the same time, the strengths and weaknesses of the parts. In other words, he's trained himself how to really *see*. Unfettered by preconceived notions, he has the skills to bring a woman's beautiful uniqueness forward. As the talented master of illusion, he can create beauty where the truth falls just a little short (or long) of the desired end.

This book will show every woman how to do the same.

9

ON MEG F. SCHNEIDER

Meg Schneider was born and raised in New York City. She attended undergraduate school at Tufts University, and received a master's degree in Counseling Psychology from Columbia University. She is a free-lance editor and writer and the author of several nonfiction books for young adult and adult audiences.

Ms. Schneider currently lives in Riverdale, New York, with her husband, Neal Brodsky.

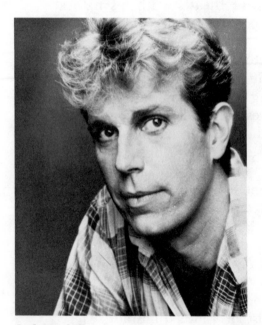 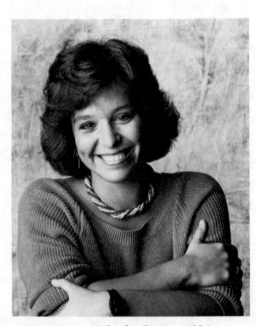

Jack Mitchell   © *Peter Tenzer/Wheeler Pictures 1984*

Introduction

Few women face the mirror with unqualified satisfaction. Whether the self-doubt is born of inner troubles or simply of an overly critical eye, a desire to improve, to do away with the negative and enhance the positive, is common.

Until now troublesome features have fallen into two categories: those that can be camouflaged with a touch of makeup, and those in need of a cosmetic surgeon's artistry. *Special Features* will blur that distinction.

I've long felt the need for a book that gets down to makeup basics—minus the glitz, minus the gossip about the author's celebrity clients, and most important, minus the promises of sudden magic transformations.

One thing is certain about the art of makeup: there's no magic about it. It involves the careful analysis of one's face and features, decisions about what to play up and what to play down, an educated selection of products and color, and a knowledgeable flexibility when it comes to application. That's the knowledge I have acquired in my twenty-three years of work in theater and film, and that is the information this book will offer.

I want to give every woman the skills to correct any problems she perceives in her face, and the power to project the look with which she is most comfortable. By creatively using light, shadow, and gracefully applied line, her problem features can enjoy a beautiful transformation. Any troublesome contour will seem to vanish as new, more pleasing, and complimentary lines emerge. The result? A flatteringly natural and unique look.

In the first part of the book, I explain the principles behind the foundations of my craft: color and shading. I cover such basics as makeup tools, color selection, and the cosmetic products you will need.

The heart of the book, however, focuses on special features: the ones that are most frequently troublesome for women, the ones they can't ignore. It seems that no matter how attractive or interesting or memorable the *combination* of features, the total effect is often missed when a woman gazes into the mirror. Instead, it's the bump in the nose, the too full lips, the receding chin that capture her critical eye. These features (which a woman may consider imperfections but which are, after all, simply the unique contours of her face) can easily make her self-conscious about her looks. This book counteracts such negative feelings by giving you *control*. Using the techniques it teaches, you can restructure and redefine any problem feature time and again.

I'm not interested in showing you how to create a glamorous mask. I'm not interested in dramatic "makeovers" that leave you looking like someone else. I'm all for giving a woman the tools to add whatever pizzazz she'd like, but I've designed this book to give her the chance to be a naturally gorgeous version of who *she* is. That's what I do in my work. I like to think that's why I continue to work. I help my clients bring their "real" character to life— whether it's their own or that of the role they are playing.

And that is why I think this book is different from all other makeup books. I feel it has a unique focus which is right in keeping with my view of beauty.

Beauty is at once a complex and yet simple thing, and the techniques I offer here reflect that fact. There is a lot to know, but the facts are easy to understand and even simpler to apply. I do not merely offer instructions, I explain what is behind them, because I do believe that in order to use my techniques well, a woman must know how and why they work. *Special Features* defines and shows, and it reflects my complete devotion to the feeling that a woman is at her most beautiful when she looks the most natural.

A PERSPECTIVE ON BEAUTY

Notions of what is beautiful in a woman are constantly changing. But since this prized quality is what you, the reader, are presumably after, it's important to first consider what beauty really is in the first place. Whenever I consult with a new client, this kind of analysis is a crucial first step, and I find that the same issues and concerns crop up again and again. Below are some of the questions I most often hear.

What Do You Think Beauty Consists Of?

I don't believe that beauty is an absolute. Beauty *is* whatever a woman feels it to be. It has to come at least in part from her inner sense of who she is and how she looks.

So much of beauty depends on things other than simply "that face." What looks breathtaking on a rainy day or in bright sunshine may not seem quite as striking in another setting. Then, too, how a woman thinks she looks, how she feels, where she is, and who she's with all play a part in her quality of beauty.

I really don't have a philosophy of beauty. Mine wouldn't matter anyway. It's the *woman's* ideas, philosophy, and feelings about herself that count. No one else's views are important.

Can You Make Me Beautiful?

My first response to this question—a very frequent question, I might add—is to laugh a little to myself. It reminds me of a cartoon I once saw depicting a young woman sitting in a chair in a beauty shop. Her hairdresser has his scissors poised in midair; his face bears a quizzical look. The caption reads, "I don't care what you do, just as long as it looks 'spring.' "

When a client says, "Make me beautiful," I react with the same bewilderment. My experience has proved that for a client to let me take over completely won't do her or me any good. So I say to her, "What is beauty for you?" If that question doesn't elicit the kind of information I need, I ask, "Why aren't you beautiful?" Women usually know what it is they don't like about their faces. They also know what they think is attractive. These things must be identified before I begin.

Once I have an idea of what troubles her, and what kind of look she would like to achieve, and what I see in *and* about her face, I go to it. I *can* usually give a woman what she wants. This is not conceit, it is fact. Any woman can look the way she feels beauty is for her, if she is open to variations. She must understand that to change her hair to blond is fine, but that the best shade for her might not be quite what she had in mind. She can have full, sensuous lips but not the exact shape of those of a particular model.

Any woman can have some version of what she's looking for. If she has a secret desire, she's already halfway to achieving it. At least part of any look comes from inside.

Is There Such a Thing as the "Perfect Face?"

My entire career is based on the fact that I believe there is, objectively, no such thing as a perfect face. It comes down to what beauty is for you.

Naturally there are some characteristics that most people find pretty. A delicate nose is an example. You might think, "well, that's always pretty, isn't it?" I'd have to say yes, in isolation, but the *effect* it has depends on the rest of the face.

Anyway, we could draw up a list of so called "ideal" features, or a list of the most exquisite faces in the world, but somewhere you'll find someone who will say, "No. That's not so great." And for him or her that judgment will be right.

"Perfection" is something that simply never crosses my mind when I look at a woman's face. In fact the word has meaning for me only in terms of achieving my goals. I wish to practice my craft to perfection. But my goal for the woman is to bring out the beauty in what she already has, to minimize the weaknesses, and to establish her *own unique* style.

As far as I know, there is no scale that measures perfection. And I'm glad of it!

Isn't Beauty Largely a Matter of Balance?

Beauty does have to do with balance: but good balance, graceful balance, interesting balance, not simply perfect balance. It's certainly true that balance is a more absolute thing than beauty. It can be measured by the eye with a certain amount of objectivity. But even this quality can sometimes serve a woman best when the features play off of one another in a tantalizing way, rather than in an even, symmetrical, and clean manner.

In fact, it's this ability to see the way in which features work together that is so very important when you devise your makeup plan. A lovely, complementary balance can be achieved with illusions, and as a result, a disproportionate element, such as a wide nose, can seem more fitting. Sometimes simply drawing attention to one feature over another by adding new lines and planes will do the trick. This is called "facial contouring." Through the use of light and shadow, an element of the face may come forward or recede or even seem to take on a new shape or contour. Success depends on the way in which you use the illusions together.

Beauty isn't simply a question of the features, separate and apart from each other. You get the whole story only when you take a look at the entire face. *Then* you can begin to work with the parts to create a lovely image.

What Distinguishes the "Interesting" Feature From the "Flawed" Feature?

In terms of how I work, the interesting feature is one I would *use*, and the flawed feature is one I would attempt to hide; that's the bottom line. Of course, how we come to label any one feature as flawed is a complicated issue, and it is also an extremely important one.

Many women move too fast. They see something they don't like, try to change it with no regard for the rest of their face, and end up drawing attention away from their best points and toward their weakest points.

I am always prepared to accept that a feature is flawed if the woman has a deep conviction about it. It may not be a problem in the eyes of anyone else, but if it's a problem for her, then it fits my definition of a flawed feature. The solution can be either to work with it or to work with the other features in such a way as to change the character of that one feature. A "flawed" feature can turn into an "interesting" or "beautiful" one quite quickly, if you deal with it appropriately.

How Can I Evaluate My Own Face and Features Objectively?

Take your time, look at everything, and follow these three steps:

First, be tolerant with the flaw. It's easy to dismiss a big nose as hateful or to be disdainful of small eyes, but it's destructive to view things in such a negative way. There may be something quite fabulous in the structure of that nose. There might be a naturally dramatic quality to those eyes. You'll miss those points if you judge too quickly.

Second, don't look in the mirror deadpan. All you'll see is a mask. Talk to yourself, laugh, study yourself from all angles. Features *do* change with the myriad expressions people wear on their faces; sparkles emerge and contours appear. Try to look at yourself as *you* really are in the world: animated, complex, and finally, attractive.

Third, as part of your attempt to find what you might want to correct, look for what you like and would love to enhance. As I mentioned before, correcting a flaw sometimes means building up something else. This approach will help you keep a balanced perspective on what your face is all about (which will also lift your spirits), and will serve to help you downplay a troublesome feature when the real solution lies with the enhancement of another one.

How Should I Approach Fads in Makeup and Makeup Techniques?

The biggest danger with fad makeup techniques is that they are fashioned to reflect the times, not the woman. Often the bright colors, creative shapes, and utter pizzazz of new fads are rather interesting. But most of the time they have nothing to do with enhancing a woman's face. They serve instead as a kind of decoration. And they can be as inappropriate for her kind of beauty as a Christmas tree would be at a Halloween party.

I do not mean to be completely negative about the new looks which continually emerge. They are attractive to many because frequently they do have a lovely and provocative flair. It gets down to a point I made earlier: A woman needs to take the current style and make it her own. She needs to adapt it to her own special features, modifying it to bring out her best, and minimizing what she likes the least. Bright red lips on one face might be absolutely striking. But on a woman whose most troublesome feature is a pair of too full lips, such a daring slash of color could work against her.

Fads can be fine as long as a woman remains as interested in what the technique or style does to her face as she is in the fashion itself. The trouble starts when she becomes so intent on achieving "the look" that she doesn't stop to consider whether it fits her face or not. First there is the face, and then comes the look; not the other way around.

Is Your Work on Stage and Screen Transferable to the Woman Who is Not in the Spotlight?

Film and stage technology today is such that an actress can wear her makeup during the filming or performance almost exactly as she would on the street. Continuing advances in lighting and film quality have given us this freedom. Naturally we sometimes go for a "bigger than life" quality, but when we do, it's deliberate. It's supposed to be seen as dramatic. Otherwise, the same beauty techniques apply, as does the principle I discussed before: that beauty is whatever a woman feels it to be. If an actress feels a certain way about herself, then it will come across. My job is to help her get there.

My work is made very rewarding, because notions of what is beautiful are now so flexible. Gone are the days of cookie-cutter beauty. Decades ago Hollywood was in the business of creating a universal, limited concept of beauty. In the thirties and forties, women flocked to plastic surgeons begging for the Myrna Loy upturned nose. Joan Crawford's severe but dramatic lips appeared everywhere. Studio heads encouraged such deification. They were always on the lookout for the next Rita Hayworth or Carole Lombard. Even Katharine Hepburn, known for her strong-willed, tenacious grip on individuality, was given early on in her career Garbo's eye makeup and hair, Dietrich's hollow cheeks, and Crawford's mouth! These attempts at imitation didn't last for long with her, but look what we might have lost had she not become powerful enough to emerge in her own right.

Neither women nor Hollywood think that way anymore. Sure, women might see a hairstyle or a look on screen that they'd like to call their own, but that's a different matter. Today the objective is to bring out what is beautifully interesting and unique in each actress's face. There's so much freedom and creativity involved!

And here is where I see a connection between on and off screen. Today's film and stage stars *want* to carve their own niche, and *so* do women who do not spend their lives in front of a spotlight. No two women look exactly alike, nor should they want to. The real beauty lies in what they see as special in themselves, and how they allow it to make a statement.

These are the questions I am frequently asked by friends and clients alike. They reflect every woman's concerns and expectations. But for readers of this book, still another question will probably loom large.

I have heard time and again that the detailed makeup instructions found in magazines don't seem to work when applied with a woman's own hand. It's important and fair to ask if my book can conquer this problem. My answer is a qualified but resounding "*yes!*" The reader must participate creatively herself. Her success will depend on how she "reads" the information in this book. The attitude with which it is taken is at least as important as what it says.

First, no two features are alike, even though they may be labeled the same. Small eyes can be small in very different ways. Full lips can come in lots of shapes, and wide noses can be constructed with all kinds of contours. Any book that proposes to state the ultimate, specific answer to *your* problem is either not telling the truth or is so thick, you'd need a crane to get it out of the bookstore.

You may have small eyes, but you certainly have them in your own unique way. The basic principles behind makeup application for each problem in this book will work only if you keep your mind free. You need to see what's going on with your face, not just the features and faces on these pages, and you need to take what this book suggests and make it your own. The most important basics are here, but every piece of advice in this book may need just a bit of adjusting to bring out the special beauty in your look. That is why simply looking up the solution to one flaw may not be enough. Each problem holds something new to learn. The solution to your particular troublesome feature may lie in combining several techniques described in this book.

Second, in terms of attitude, perseverance is the key. As I said earlier, this business of makeup application isn't magic. There are many beauty and makeup books out there that use the word *magic* in their titles. It's as if people believe, or at least want to believe, that with just a quick flick of the wrist a true beauty is born. It doesn't happen that way, and it's actually just as well. Experimenting with makeup can be wonderful fun! But it will only be enjoyable if your expectations are realistic. It would be tragic if you threw up your hands in distress in the first unsuccessful five minutes! I apply makeup for a living, and I always have to experiment with my clients' faces before resolving a problem for both of us. Why shouldn't you?

It's critically important when using this book to keep in mind what you know about your own face. Being aware of your own special features will help you to identify your problem and adapt the techniques you can use. This takes time, confidence, and patience.

Special Features is not gospel! It is a guide. Ultimately you do have to make your own way. But this book will help you stay on the right path.

PART ONE
PREPARATION

1
SKIN CARE

Everything in this book rests both figuratively and literally on the surface of the skin. It is easy, therefore, to see why you must establish a regular skin care routine. Not only can the skin be harmed by the products you apply, but it can also actually affect the look of the makeup itself. It is an extraordinarily sensitive organ, and it is also very individual. So I encourage you to make use of the many products available for early morning and nighttime cleansing and moisturizing.

In this chapter and throughout the book, I refrain from recommending specific products simply because so many excellent ones are available and I don't wish to stop the reader from trying any of them. The people behind the cosmetic counters can act as your consultants. These individuals aren't just sales forces: they've been trained in their products by the cosmetic company and are usually quite knowledgeable. If you have doubts or don't want to risk making expensive mistakes, ask for small tester kits containing one or two applications of each product in a given line.

Aside from the importance of keeping your skin in top condition simply for the beautiful and healthful benefits it brings, it is also important to work out a skin care routine specifically geared toward makeup application. This is what I will cover here.

CLEANSERS

You can use top-of-the-line products (lotions and cream cleansers) or simple mild soap and water. What really matters is that you *completely* remove the old layers of makeup before you move to apply new ones. Otherwise, the skin could begin to suffocate, manifesting problems that would require a doctor's care.

Cleansers come in the form of solid and liquid soaps, lotions, and creams. They dissolve makeup and remove excess oils that can clog pores. Dry skin may do better with lotion soaps, while oily skin could benefit more from mild solid soaps. After you have worked the cleanser into the classic trouble spots (around the nose, under the eyes, back to the ears, and in the crease of the chin), wash off thoroughly with tepid water.

A cold rinse to help close pores, followed by a gentle drying with a clean, *dry* towel, using a patting motion, will leave your skin feeling refreshed.

TONERS

Toners can also be labeled fresheners or astringents. They can be very mild (with no alcohol) for sensitive skin, or stronger (with alcohol), often necessary for oily skin. Toners remove excess oils and residue from cleansers, and they stimulate the skin, bringing the blood "up" for a healthier appearance. They close the pores, creating that pleasant "tightening" feeling.

Remember to use your toner with a fresh cotton ball, not a tissue. Tissues are made of wood pulp which has tiny splinters that can irritate your face. The soft absorbent quality of the cotton ball will be much kinder to your skin.

MOISTURIZERS

The skin is 90 percent water, and it is critically important to keep it that way. Moisturizers will help. They seal in the natural moisture of your skin, form an effective barrier between your skin and harsh weather, and create a smooth base for makeup. A light, protective film applied before you begin your makeup session will provide you with a receptive surface upon which to work.

Moisturizers vary in composition to suit the needs of different skin types. When buying these products in the store, consult the salesperson to find out which are meant for your skin type. Cleansers and moisturizers are meant to work together, so it is a good idea to stay with *one* product line. Each cosmetic company has developed its package as a complete skin care regimen.

FACIAL HAIR

After you use cleansers, toners, and moisturizers to prepare the face for makeup, you should take the final step and clear the skin of the facial hair which could work against your beauty goals. In order for the cosmetics to seem part of the skin instead of resting on top of it, the surface of the face should be absolutely smooth.

Excessive facial hair on the cheeks can easily be bleached. The mustache can either be bleached or waxed. Your decision on which is best for you should depend on the sensitivities of your skin and the goals you might have for your lip makeup. If the hair is very thick you may want to simply wax it off—even a light blond mustache can be quite noticeable. If you are trying to redefine or slightly thicken the upper lip, the pencil color could bleed into the hair, creating an uneven line. The same principle applies to light blonde eyebrows. Without a cleanly waxed arch, it is difficult to apply shadows smoothly to the eye area. If these extremes don't apply to you, you may not have to do a thing. Light facial hairs usually won't cause any problems.

NOTE: If you opt to use a professional for either the bleaching or waxing procedures, have your eyelashes dyed at the same time. Most people's lashes are a few shades lighter than their hair color. Darkening the lashes will give them the same drama that a heavy application of mascara lends, without the flaking, sticking, and running. Once you have this darker base, you merely have to add the mascara for a light shaping, lengthening, or thickening.

2
THE KIT

In my work as a makeup artist, I aim for a soft and natural look. My makeup kit reflects this. It includes tools, cosmetics, and colors that will work together to create a polished look that is both simple and flattering. Whether you opt for a dramatic style or a subtle flair, that is up to you. If you tend to apply makeup with a light touch (as I do), the techniques in this book will give your face a quiet glow. Aggressively used, the suggestions could lead to a more forceful and glamorous statement. Either way, everything you will need is here. And it's important to note that your makeup kit needn't stop where this one does.

I said earlier that I don't favor fad makeup styles that are imitated without regard to the individual face. But I do want to make it clear that if adapted correctly, the looks *can* be fun and effective. By "correctly" I mean:

- taking into consideration your own features;
- experimenting with colors and styles;
- being open to the limitations your face may impose on the look you are after;
- applying the highly stylized makeup *over* your basic makeup.

Feel free to play with the fashionable approaches, but use them as extra touches to your normal daily makeup. By doing this you will add style to an already balanced look, not simply an exotic and sometimes unflattering edge to an unfinished look.

The application of makeup ought to be fun. Individual approaches to the sequence of steps, the work area, and even tools and

27

cosmetic products are absolutely allowed, even advisable. The best makeup job is done by the woman who applies her makeup in her own way—with ease and confidence.

This chapter will give you what you need to know in order to proceed. The information in this section does follow a sequence of sorts. Foundation comes before highlighting and contouring. But the rest is up to you.

TOOLS

Any tool works best if it is well made. Quality tools last longer than poor ones, do the job they are supposed to do, and rarely create new problems. Do take this into consideration when visiting the cosmetic counter. There is a wide range of products and a wide range of prices. The most expensive is not always the best, so use your eye and seek the advice of the salesperson before you make a decision.

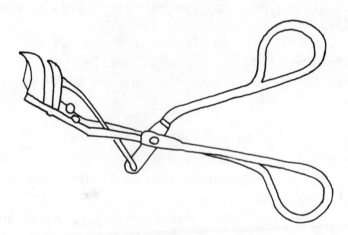

Eyelash Curler

This is an essential tool. At first it may be a bit difficult to get used to, but it will lend a wonderful, natural drama to the lashes. Use it directly before applying mascara. Place the curler at the base of the lashes, and gently squeeze, holding for a moment. The lashes will turn up gracefully.

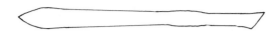

Tweezers

This tool should be capable of firmly grasping and smoothly pulling out the unwanted hair. It can be found in a pointed, straight, and slanted design. The choice is yours. I prefer the slanted-tip construction as the angle seems to work well in my hand.

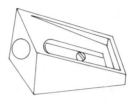

Pencil Sharpener

You can't make do without this. Regular sharpeners are not designed for makeup pencils and will only ruin the pencil. These special sharpeners come in two different sizes so be sure you select the correct one for your pencils. Don't try for razor-tip points. If the point is too sharp, round it off! Nothing in my makeup technique demands a crisp, fine, sharp line.

Brushes

Fine brushes are crucial to smooth and natural-looking makeup application. The length and width of the handle is up to you. Don't hesitate to spend a little time in the store holding them in mock makeup application positions. It may be the only way you can tell if they will work for you.

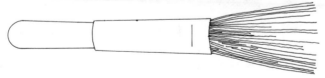

THE POWDER BRUSH: This is the biggest brush in your makeup kit. It is over an inch wide and about an inch and a half long. It is to be used for applying and removing loose and pressed powder to set makeup on the face, neck, and shoulders. The longer, thicker, and fuller the brush, the better!

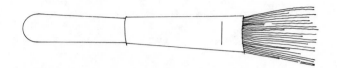

THE POWDER ROUGE BRUSH AND THE POWDER CON-TOUR BRUSH: I use identical brushes for rouge and contour powders. The brush I use is about three-quarters of an inch wide and about three-quarters of an inch to an inch long. It fans out slightly at the top and tapers off into a flat dimension toward the center. It should be *very* soft. Sometimes contour brushes can be stiff and blunt, and thus tend to leave a concentration of color instead of a softer shading. It is important that the rouge and contour powders blend into the face instead of simply sitting on the surface.

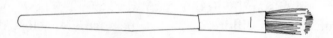

THE SMALLER POWDER SHADING BRUSH: This brush is approximately half an inch wide with bristles that are three-quarters of an inch to an inch long. It is used to blend powder and shadows around the eyelid, and under the eye. (The sponge applicators which often come with shadows will do the same, though I prefer Q-tips or this smaller powder brush.)

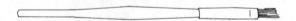

THE SHADOW BRUSH: This small brush has a nice weight to it and can be used for both cream and powder. It is cut on the bias, and tapered down so the end point can reach the inner corner of the eye. It's approximately an eighth of an inch wide with a blunt surface at the top to facilitate blending. This brush is commonly used on the upper and lower lid as well as for contouring the nose and under the lower lip. It can be used for many colors, but must be washed thoroughly before switching tones.

THE LIP BRUSH: This brush with its tapered end and flat center gives you the ability to make precise corrections. Look for one with a nice clean shape and firmness. The tip can be used for outlining, and the flat side for applying color and lip gloss.

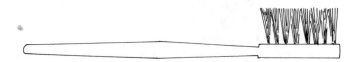

THE EYEBROW AND EYELASH BRUSH: Used to shape eyebrows and separate lashes after applying mascara, this is a brittle brush made of stiff natural fiber which usually has two rows and looks like a thin toothbrush.

Q-TIPS: These are indispensible, in my opinion. They are a clean, sanitary way of putting on powdered eye shadows, smudging eyeliner or shadows, and removing little mistakes such as spots of mascara on the cheeks.

Lighting

When it comes to lighting, in my opinion it is useless to try to describe the perfect place for makeup application. There really is no such situation, if only because people are seen in many different kinds of light. One "perfect" lighting situation may not mean a thing when a woman proceeds to move around her world.

The important thing is for a woman to find a comfortable place with a nonglaring light in which to work. Whether she sits cross-legged on the floor or works over the bathroom sink, it makes little difference as long as she has enough time and space to easily control the brushes and pencils in her hand. In fact, the only error in lighting and location a woman could make is to finish her makeup in front of one mirror, turn off the light, pick up her bag, and walk out the door without a second glance. Big mistake! As I said before, you will be seen in all kinds of light throughout the day. It's critical that you check your makeup in other mirrors and lighting situations before leaving the house. By doing so you will get a true feel for your look and will allow yourself the opportunity to make adjustments.

MAKEUP

The general approach to makeup application is an individual one. Other than the fact that foundation (if you use it) should be applied to the face first, and the contouring shading and highlighting next, the sequence is up to you. Whatever makes the experience relaxing and enjoyable is what counts. Of course common sense must rule (blusher shouldn't go under highlighter), but it would be dishonest of me to insist that one system is better than the next.

The chapters in Part II are arranged in accordance with my suggested sequence. But as always, you can make the routine your own. If you have a highlighter in your hand, doing away with laugh lines and highlighting the area under your brow at the same time could work well for you. Working layer on layer, rather than feature to feature, will see you finished sooner. But in order for this system to be good for you, it may take time. The more familiar you are with your new makeup techniques, the easier it will be to take an expedient route.

You'll notice that of all the makeup colors, the ones I most often prescribe for contouring and shadowing are shades of taupe. Why is this color so versatile? When light shines on the face, the color of the shadows is taupe. Therefore, when you use a taupe makeup, you are in fact recreating the color of shadow on the skin. The effect is completely natural. You almost won't know that you are wearing makeup, and yet you can seem to change the shape of your features! In addition, the shades of taupe will work for any complexion because they mix naturally with all skin colors. If you have pale skin, simply use the shade sparingly. Darker skin will take a heavier concentration of color.

Here is the collection of makeup I think it's most important to have on hand.

SPECIAL COLORS

These are my colors. I use these highly special tones to achieve a finely contoured yet natural look. For this reason, you will not find the rainbow of
colors that you might at a department store counter. This section on special
colors is designed to help you understand the advice throughout the book.
Experiment with these makeups. Give yourself the time to learn the power
of these tones. It is startling to see how easily a tawny or rose blush can
straighten a nose.

Once you've mastered these skills, go out and create the color palette
that is best for you. This is your base. Pursue the rainbow later.

PRIMARY USES:
Smooth furrowed brow
Hide smile lines
Erase under-eye shadows
Used with contouring
     makeup to sculpt nose,
     cheeks, and neck.

CONCEALING
HIGHLIGHTER

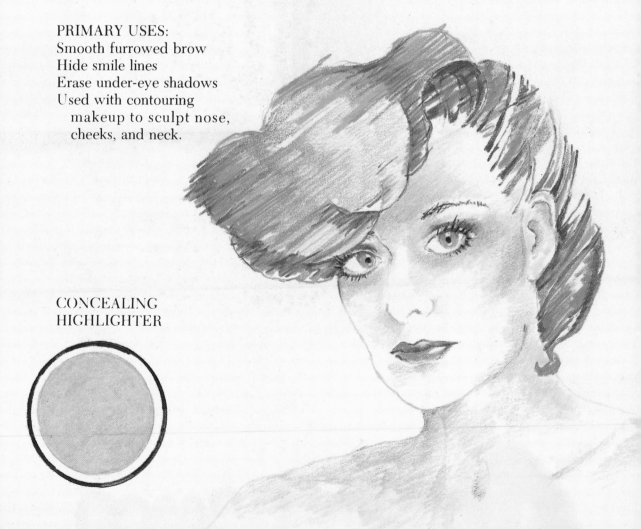

PRIMARY USES:

Shade eye area
Bring out cheekbones
Sculpt nose, chin, and neck

Hide skin imperfections
Set the foundation and
  contouring makeup
Give your look a natural soft
  finish

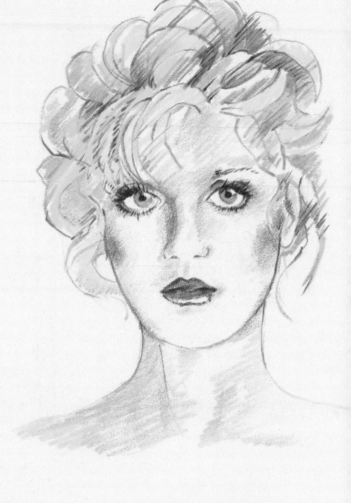

DEEP CONTOURING CREAM

TAUPE CONTOURING CREAM AND POWDER

LOOSE POWDER

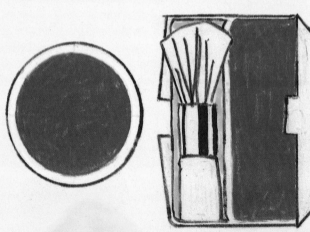

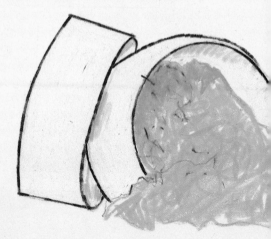

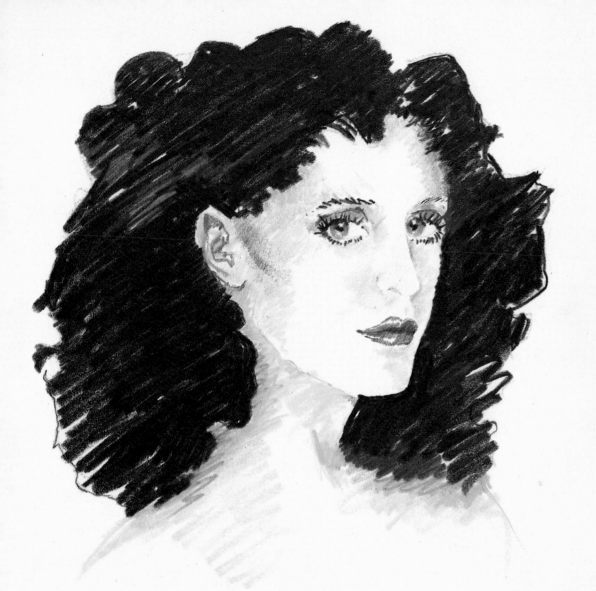

BLUSHER

Rose   Tawny

PRIMARY USES:
Color cheeks
Sculpt forehead

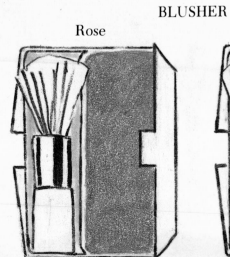

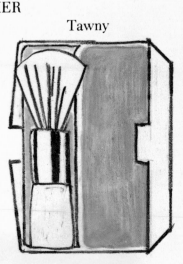

EYE SHADOW

Earth Tones   Jewel Tones

PENCILS

Pink/White   Charcoal Brow

Taupe   Black

Sienna   Red

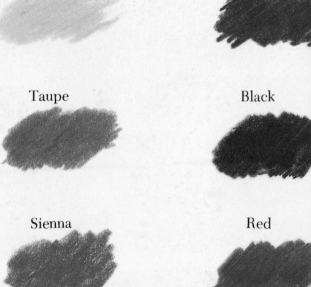

Foundations

The first question you must ask yourself is "Do I really need it?" All of the makeup suggested in this book can be applied on top of moisturizer. If your answer is "no," then just move right on to the contouring makeup. If it's a hesitant, "Well, in some places I do," then apply foundation accordingly. You may only need it in the T-area between the eyes, down the nose, and around the mouth. The less on the skin, the better. However, if you feel you do need the foundation to even out your skin color, it should be applied as sheerly as possible.

When shopping for a foundation that is right for you, test the color on your face, your jaw, and the insides of your wrists. (Be sure to test *over* a moisturizer. That is how you will be applying it at home. Since moisturizers can cause a slight change in the color, it's important to see what that change will be.)

In terms of color do not try to change your skin color dramatically. Instead, go for a slightly different tone. A sallow skin can use a slightly rosy foundation. A ruddy complected person may do better with a beige color to soften the red.

NOTE: Don't be afraid to mix colors if you can't seem to find the one that's right for you. Ask the salesperson for a little help.

Contouring Colors

HIGHLIGHTERS: Highlighting is used to bring an area forward, and to erase the shadows a concave area can create.

I find that highlighter creams work better than liquids, sticks, and powders, because they are easier to blend with the fingertips or brush. The color should not be too pink, white, or yellow. Choose a highlighter two or three shades lighter than your base for the most subtle and natural effects (see chart).

TAUPE CONTOUR CREAM AND POWDER: Throughout this book I discuss contouring: creating lines, shadows, and other dramatic and attractive dimensions with contouring creams or powder. For the more subtle definitions specified in the upcoming chapters, the powder or cream can be used interchangeably (see chart).

DEEP CONTOUR CREAM: The deep tone is used in areas where we need the stronger control of a cream in a limited way. Powders and lighter creams work well for a softer definition, while the deeper creams, a very concentrated makeup, create a more powerful and specific contour (see chart).

POWDERS: Powders are a wonderful, problem-solving companion to facial makeup. They soften or hide imperfections in the skin, help to blend the edges of the contouring colors, and most important, they set the foundation and contouring creams and powders, giving the skin a radiant sheen.

A loose, translucent powder which adds no color (though it may appear white in its package) lightly brushed onto the face, neck, and shoulders will give your look a natural soft finish. It must, however, be very carefully and evenly applied. After dipping your big brush into the powder make sure to shake the brush in order to get rid of the excess before stroking the powder onto your face. Begin under the eyes, move to the cheekbones, forehead, eyelids, and nose, and finish off with the chin, jaw, neck, and shoulders.

A pressed translucent powder patted on throughout the day will serve as a good touch-up, virtually assuring you that the makeup you applied that morning stays fresh, not to mention "put!"

And once again, the loose translucent or pressed translucent powder can be used without a foundation. Moisturizer may be all you need.

BLUSHERS: Blushers can be used both for adding healthful color as well as for soft contouring and accenting. Since most people use this makeup for both, it's especially important that the color seem natural. Otherwise the "painted doll" effect is all you will get. Form, and a little tone know-how, help.

I prefer a cake blusher as opposed to a cream, especially if I'm using a contouring color (highlighter or taupe). This is because the cream blush could mix with the contouring makeup, ruining the intended effect. However, if you are not using any facial contouring techniques, certainly the cream blusher can give an excellent and natural-looking color. It *must* be applied smoothly, and carefully blended into the skin.

Real-life blush, the kind you get after a quick jog on a winter's day, is actually blood showing through the particular tones of your skin. The blush you choose should reflect that same color. Bright fluorescents or pale pastels simply won't give you a natural rich, deep, glow.

I use two basic tones (see chart):

Rose: These tones are good for the ashy or light beige skin color which needs a touch of brightness.

Tawny: These tones are excellent for women with ruddy complexions. They will soften the redness and yet still leave a healthy sparkle.

Everyone's skin reflects a unique combination of tones. Despite the classic efforts to categorize the colors, such as "olive" or "ivory," the truth remains that within each category there can be huge differences which should and will affect the color blush you wear.

Be sure then to experiment at the makeup counter. Sweep on a bit of blush. Walk around and look in different mirrors under different lighting. And remember, you're after that "just been jogging" look!

Pencils

The pencils listed here can be used both for contouring as well as simple coloration. They appear throughout the following chapters and most are useful in many different ways.

Pink–White: for use as a highlighter

Taupe: for eyebrows, eyeliner, shadowing, and shading of nose and eyes

Sienna: for eyebrows, contouring and coloring lips, and shading eyes

Charcoal Brown: for eyebrows and eyeliner

Black: for eyebrows and eyeliner

Red: for use as a lip liner or lipstick pencil.

The pencils should be soft enough to blend easily. But these pencils also must be firm enough so that the colors they produce don't run or bleed. A "medium soft" texture is just right. A good way to check for "feel" before purchasing is to simply touch the point of the pencil (they always come sharpened) with your fingertip. If it has a little give it's probably fine. Too much or too little will get you into trouble.

Eyeshadows

Eyeshadows can be a wonderful accent for the eye. They can lend definition (yes, contours!), bring out the best in your eye and skin color, and generally impart a delicious sparkle to your look. But as always, I recommend the subtle application of a subtle color, usually some shade of taupe.

It's also important to keep in mind that your decision as to which color to wear should *not* be solely dependent on your "coloring." Shadows can have very significant effects on a face, and thus you should consider the structural elements as well, before whipping out that sky-blue shadow. A dash of color around the eye can just as easily point out the problems as it can enhance the assets.

Throughout the chapter on eyes, I mention shadows, creams, and powders, and the ways in which they can be used to minimize a flaw and maximize the rest. Briefly, cream tends to give more intense color than powder, offering a strong, specific definition. Powders can be easier to blend and offer a gentler accent. Brushes, Q-tips, or the fingertip are all useful as applicators, each offering different amounts of control depending on the user. You will have to assess what works the best for you.

I view the colors that are available in two categories: earth and jewel (see chart). In each I suggest the more subtle tones as I find that gently applied they will seem like part of the face, instead of simply "window dressing."

Also, keep in mind that the taupe contouring cream or powder and deep contouring cream can be used to shadow the eyes, when my instructions call for shadowing in these colors.

Mascara

I use only two colors, black or brown. The kind of mascara you choose, regular, waterproof, or with fibers, is up to your individual preference, requirements, and your personal chemistry.

Waterproof mascara is good if you have a problem with smudging, though the remover you may need to use could be troublesome for sensitive eyes. Fibered mascara is excellent for thin lashes, though it could be a problem for those who wear contact lenses. Regular mascara is perfect for full lashes which need just a light shaping and coloring.

Aside from the specific tips on application in Chapter 5, here are some general points to remember:

- Make sure you cover each lash from top to bottom. First, move the tip of the brush horizontally across the lashes as close to the base as possible; then sweep the wand in an upward motion.
- Use the eyelash brush to separate the lashes for a more even and natural look.
- Mascara is very drying. Use a gentle eye cream after removing the makeup. It will moisten and clean.

Finally, *do not* keep the wand mascara for more than three months. There are tiny bacteria on your lashes that will stay on your wand and then find their way into the tube where they will grow. Even if you've only used the mascara once or twice, *throw it out* after three months. Otherwise you could find yourself with "irritating" eye problems.

Lipsticks

The question of color is usually the biggest issue here. And the answer is the same as it was for selecting the proper blusher. You will want to find a color that looks natural: that reflects the feeling of blood showing through the skin.

The sienna and red pencils I mentioned earlier will work for almost anyone. They can be used in combination with clear or tinted lip gloss or a lipstick that closely matches your own lip color. (If your lips are very pale a simple exploration at a makeup counter will help you find a color that matches what you would like to call your own. But again, check more than one mirror!) There is an array of glosses and lips colors that will afford you a natural look.

The information and color chart in this section will provide you with the basic tools and makeup to achieve the look I always work toward. The key word is *natural*, both in terms of color and application. For it's not enough that you purchase the right things. You have to use them in a way that will lend you a healthy and lovely glow.

Part II will show you how to do this.

PART TWO
SPECIAL FEATURES

3
FACIAL LINES AND SHADOWS

Goal: This first step in makeup application serves both to bring forward receding areas and to camouflage shadows. The highlighting techniques described here will impart a look of smoothness and light.

The Most Classic Error: Never use stark white as a highlighter. It won't hide the lines. Its unnatural appearance will only draw attention to the flaw you are trying to cover up by making the area look swollen. Also, the shadows may turn gray soon after application.

FURROWED BROW

Horizontal and vertical lines and folds form in between the brows.

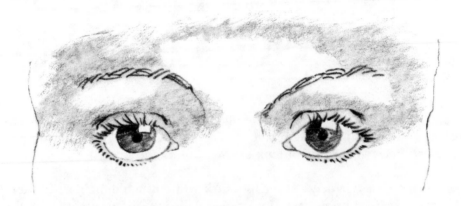

Select a highlighter that is a little lighter than your natural skin tone. Apply the color gently between the brows, onto the forehead, and down over the bridge of the nose. Blend the highlighter in evenly so that there is no clearly definable line where the color and your natural skin tone meet.

Glamour Tip: Apply a little highlighter directly under the arch of the eyebrow, accentuating the natural curve. The eyes will seem to lighten up.

Classic Error: No matter what the facial line or shadow, never use a pearlessence highlighter. It will only spotlight the problem.

DEEPLY FURROWED BROW

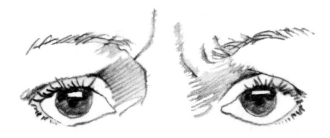

Step 1. Lightly blend in a little highlighter.

Step 2. Using a light pink pencil, draw a line directly into the furrows. Blot the color lightly, but do not blend in the pencil.

Classic Error: The pink pencil only works for vertical furrow lines. Attempting to camouflage horizontal creases with the pencil will add stripes, not smoothness, to your face.

SMILE LINES

Creases around the mouth and along the nasal labial fold.

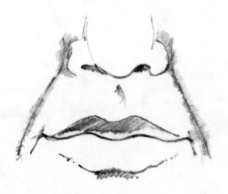

Apply a highlighter down along the smile lines if the folds are particularly deep.

Classic Error: When you apply highlighter, always strive for a sheer effect. If you stroke the color on too heavily, the lines will not disappear and will in fact be further emphasized by the "caked" look.

UNDER-EYE SHADOWS

Dark shadowy circles around the eyes create a tired appearance.

Step 1. Stroke on a highlighter under the eyes, starting along the sides of the nose near where the eyes rest and moving to the outer corners. Extend the tone lightly onto the cheek. The concentration of color should be on the darker areas, but blended down to avoid that "orb of light" look.

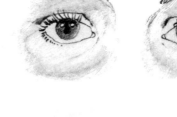

Step 2. If the shadows are very deep cover them with the pink pencil, after applying the highlighter. Do this only on the darkest areas. Blot the color carefully so that it merges smoothly with the natural skin tone. Again, never spread the pink tone.

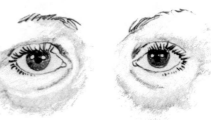

Common Error: A cream highlighter (no matter what the problem you are erasing) should never be used alone. The shine will make the area look swollen. Remember to lightly powder over the highlighter with a tone which matches the cream.

4
EYEBROWS

The eyebrows are all too frequently ignored. At best they are viewed as an issue to focus on when all else is taken care of. But this is an enormous mistake.

The eyebrow is a kind of frame for the eye. Just as one would never simply place any frame, no matter what the color, shape, or size, on a favored piece of art, so would it be wrong to approach the brow as though it is an independent entity existing only to reflect well or not at all upon itself.

A frame does have power. It can absolutely bring out the best of the thing it surrounds, effecting a remarkable change in its look. But left unattended it can also emphasize a weakness, and more tragic than that, hide a true beauty.

EYEBROWS

Goal: By following the natural shape of the eyebrow while at the same time considering the contours of the eye and the brow as a frame, any flaws will be minimized and the beauty of the whole face will be enhanced and flattered.

Tips on Shaping

- Either tweezing or waxing will work well when shaping eyebrows, though tweezing will tend to give you more control.
- Do not tweeze directly before applying your makeup as a slight swelling is bound to occur. Instead, try and make time before you go to sleep.
- Place a cube of ice on the skin right before you begin to work. It will shrink the skin, draw blood away, and desensitize the area.
- Don't completely shape one eyebrow, and then the other. Rather, move back and forth until you have achieved a clear, graceful balance.
- For very thick brows tweeze two hairs at a time from the middle of the brow. It will help to quickly thin them out. If they are still inordinately bushy and unruly, you can also brush them down, and with small scissors, trim the ends just a bit. Then brush them back into shape for a smoother, more refined look.
- If you are trying to subtly change the shape of, or thicken the brow you will find the eyebrow brush a very useful tool. By brushing the hair firmly in a particular direction, the shape will become more defined and the brow itself will seem fuller.

Tips on Coloring

- The eyebrows should be a few shades lighter than your own hair color. The softer tone tends to open out the face.
- If your brows are dark, you can lightly bleach with facial-hair bleach. Be sure to check the progress at regular intervals. You can always go back and bleach a bit more.
- If the bleaching process leaves you with a color that is too light (or if your natural color is too fair) a taupe pencil will add a richer tone

48

to the brow. Be sure the pencil is soft enough to coat the hairs with color, not shade the skin.

Below are some basic guidelines for helping you design the eyebrows that will work well for you. I have chosen to detail the brows of close-set, well-spaced, and far-apart eyes because the solutions are quite different and represent most of the options that are open to you. (I do mention these techniques briefly in the eyes chapter, as a reminder.)

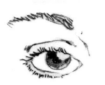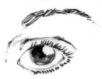

Close-set Eyes

If your eyes are too close together be sure to completely clean the area between the brows, pushing the inner corner of the brows back so that they start slightly in from the inner corners of the eyes. The center of the arch should rest a bit beyond the center of the eye, approximately aligned with the outside of the iris. Allow the outside corners of the brow to taper off subtly. Attention will be drawn outward instead of inward.

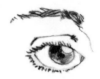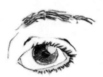

Well-spaced Eyes

Again, clean the space between the eyebrows, allowing the brow to start directly above the inner corner of the eye. The arch should be directly over the pupil of the eye, gracefully arching up and out.

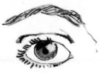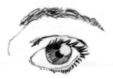

Eyes Too Far Apart

After cleaning out the space between the brows, allow the inner corner of the brow to start a bit over the inner corner of the eye. The arch should be aligned approximately with the inside curve of the iris. The outside corners of the brow should end almost directly above the outside corner of the eye. By pulling the brows closer together, the eyes will not seem so far apart.

5
THE EYES

Some people believe that because of their immediate beauty, the eyes are the first feature to capture the attention of an admirer. Then there are those who think that the eyes leave a lasting impression because of what the viewer sees in them. These people would argue that it's the unspoken message in the eyes that holds the power to hypnotize.

No matter where the truth lies, it remains that the eyes are a magnificently expressive element of the face. Enhancing their beauty with illusions of definition, size, and color will only add to the glory of what is communicated, and of what is seen in that special moment.

SMALL EYES

Seem to lack definition and are out of balance in relation to other features. Have a slight or narrow upper lid.

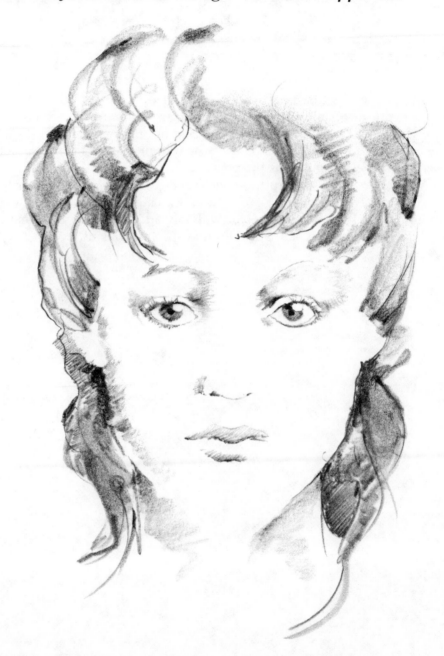

Goal: The eyes will take on a more dramatic definition through the use of light and shadow. Taupe eyeshadow playing against the natural skin tone will seem to open up the eye, creating an expressive feature and a more balanced face.

Step 1. Using a taupe shadow, cream or powder, evenly shade the upper lid up through the hood of the eye to the inner corner of brow, and down over the bone line to the outer edge of the eye. Using the same shadow, continue around underneath the eye. Blend edges with a fingertip or brush in an outward motion until you have created the desired "widening" effect.

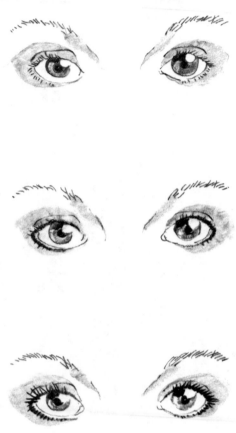

Step 2. With a darker tone blunt-tip eyeliner pencil (see chart in makeup kit for your appropriate shade), follow the line of the lid to create a soft definition. Starting at the lashes on the upper lid, follow around and under, intensifying the color in the outer edges. Dot the color into the lower lashes to create the effect of a line. Smudge with a brush or finger.

Step 3. Curl lashes with a lash curler and then apply mascara. Use a pink–white pencil along the inner lower lid. Be sure to have a well-arched brow. Lightly extend with brow pencil. Using either mascara to match your eyebrow color, or hairspray on a toothbrush, brush in an upward motion. (Some individuals are allergic to hairspray. If your skin is very sensitive, it may be wise to avoid it.)

Classic Errors: Don't use pastel blue or green shadows. They will close the eyes rather than open them. Also, don't put eyeliner inside the lower lid.

Glamour Tip: Bring the blunt pencil eyeliner up and around into the socket for a more dramatic effect, or use an even deeper-toned shadow on the lid.

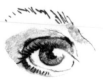

EYES TOO FAR APART

Seem set at a distance from bridge of the nose and have a floating, slightly disconnected look.

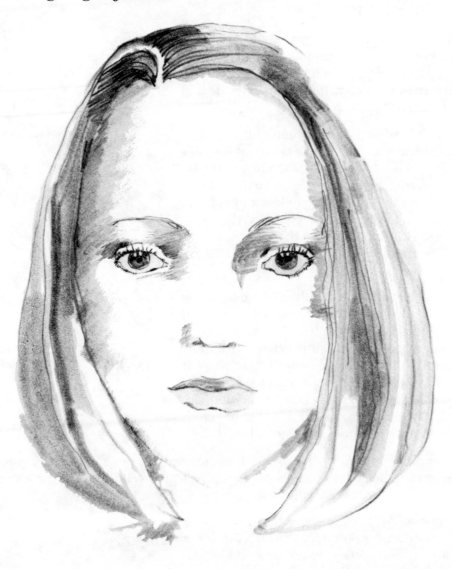

Goal: Here, the eyeshadow and eyeliner tones applied inward, instead of in an outward direction, will seem to pull the eyes closer together to create a tighter relationship between them and a stronger balance in the face.

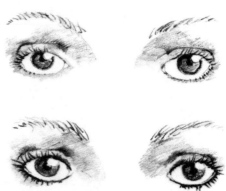

Step 1. Apply a foundation darker than your skin tone in the inner corner of the eye, up through the brow, through the lid to the socket, into the bridge of the nose, and around and under, following the contour of the eye.

Step 2. Using an eyeliner pencil, bring the color around the contour of the eye, concentrating the color on the inner corner. Carefully smudge the outer corner.

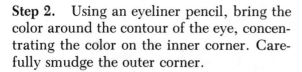

Step 3. Clean the space in between the eyebrows leaving the lines as natural as possible. Allow the eyebrow to begin closer to the bridge of the nose than the inner corner of the eye. Curl lashes and apply mascara, making sure not to stroke in an outward motion. Lashes will always tend to curl in the direction in which they grow, but you should avoid doing anything that will draw attention to the outer corners of the eye.

Classic Error: Do not extend the outer edges of the brow hoping for a more balanced look. The eyes will only seem to move even farther apart.

EYES TOO CLOSE TOGETHER

Seem to move together and rest on the inner contour of the nose.

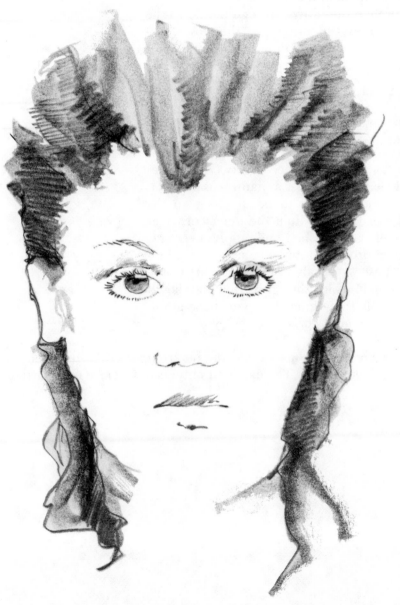

Goal: Through the use of shadows applied to attract attention "out" rather than "in," the eyes will seem to move apart, resting in more graceful balance with the hairline and the nose.

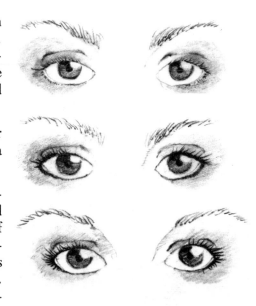

Step 1. Place a light-colored foundation on the inner corner of the eye, up to the brow. Beginning one-third of the way from the inner corner, apply a darker shadow over the lid, around and underneath the eye. Blend outwards.

Step 2. Apply a pencil liner along the outer two-thirds of the eye. Smudge gently for a subtle definition.

Step 3. Be sure to keep the space in between the brows clean. It will work toward "separating" the eyes. The inner corner of the brow should be even with the inner corner of the eye. Extend the brow outwards slightly to further create an illusion of space. Curl lashes, and apply mascara concentrating on the outer corners.

BULGING EYES

Seem to protrude out from the facial planes.

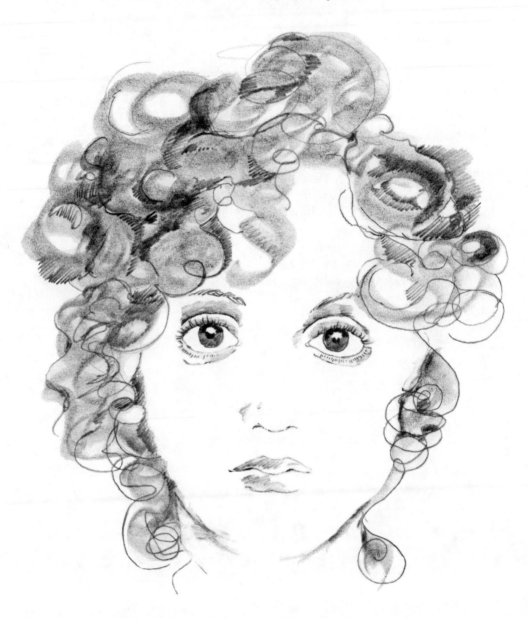

Goal: As this is a problem rooted more in dimension than shape, light and shadow will work together to create an illusion of smoother facial contours. The eyes will be simply and gently illuminated, while the bulge, lightly shadowed, begins to recede.

Step 1. Using a taupe shadow, or a tone slightly darker than your natural skin color, shade the entire hood up to and into the brow. Continue around and underneath the eye. The amount of surface below the eye that you cover with the shadow will depend completely on the degree of the problem and your own capable assessment! Just keep in mind that dark shading makes an area recede. The more pronounced the bulge, the more you'll want to shadow.

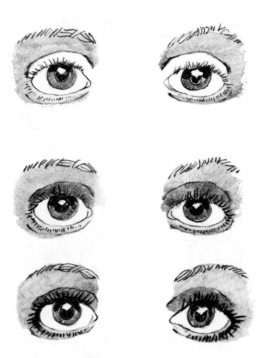

Step 2. Choose a dark eyeshadow: either a dark taupe, a deep skin tone, or a deep jewel tone. Apply this shadow to the lid and around the eye in a defined line. Blend into the lighter color.

Step 3. Apply a pencil eyeliner, starting away from the inner corner and moving around the eye. Gently smudge with fingertip.

Classic Error: Don't use light or frosted colors. The eyes will only appear to pop out further!

TURNED-DOWN EYES

*Seem to droop at the outer corner pulling the face
downward—tired looking.*

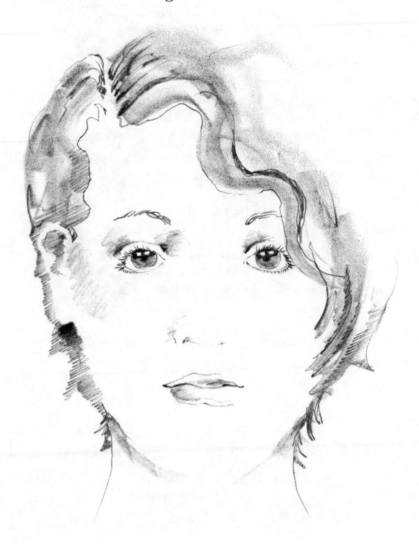

Goal: With the strategic application of warm, natural shadows, the outer corners of the eyes will seem to lift, attracting attention in an upward motion and creating a look of sparkle and light.

Step 1. Place a neutral tone or color (lavender or muted green, for example) on the eyelid. Next, choose a dark skin tone or taupe shadow. Start at the inner corner of the eye and sweep on the color above the eyelid extending it upward at the outer corner.

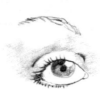 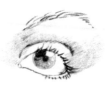

Step 2. Apply eyeliner, beginning slightly away from the inner corners of the eye, and thicken the color at the upper outside contour. Add mascara and curl.

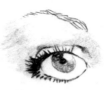 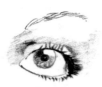

TURNED-UP EYES

Seem to fall inward creating a slightly cross-eyed look.

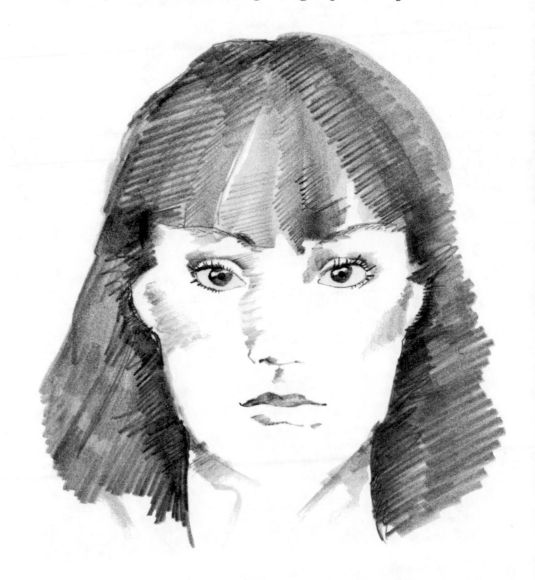

Goal: Attention will be drawn upward through the use of deeper shadows on the inside corners as a kind of lure. As a result, the eyes will appear better balanced and more in harmony with the rest of the face.

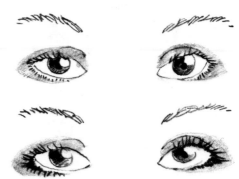

Step 1. Apply taupe shadow on the lid. Bring it up to the bone and level with the dip in the upper lid, then around and under the outer corner of the eye.

Step 2. Stroke on a trace of eyeliner starting away from the inner edges. Extend it a little past the upper outside contour, and thicken and extend in the lower outer corner. Apply mascara in an outward motion and curl.

DEEP-SET EYES

Often seem lost or hooded. Lid seems to sink back into the socket.

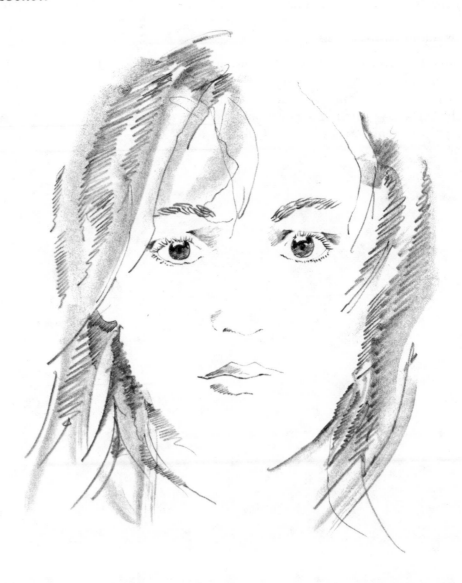

Goal: Through the use of light tones, what seems to disappear will become more noticeable; with the application of darker shadows, what appears too prominent will gently recede. The eyes will make a brighter and more openly dramatic statement.

Step 1. Place a light skin tone, taupe, or pale shadow on the lid. (Yes! Now is the time to use any subtle, light color you wish.) Starting at the eye crease or socket, apply a darker tone up toward the brow and around under the eye. This shadow can be blended out to the desired shape, depending on the natural contour of your eye.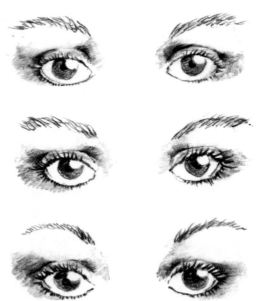

Step 2. Using a minimal amount of eyeliner pencil, add a thin line for definition along the top lid and along two-thirds of the lower lid.

Step 3. It's important to keep a clean arch, as you will want to increase the space between the eyelid and brow. Gracefully arch the brow to create as large a plane as possible, maintaining the natural shape.

Classic Error: Don't place a stark white or bright color on the lid. It will serve to move that area out, but the rest of the eye will seem to sink into oblivion!

Don't apply heavy eyeliner. Too much "definition" on a deep-set eye will close it right up.

Glamour Tip: Using the rouge you apply to your cheeks, highlight under the brow, blending into the brow line for a lovely brightening effect.

6
THE NOSE

The nose is perhaps the most conspicuous feature on the face, and it is often the owner's least favorite one because it is indeed a feature that is frequently and rigidly judged at "face value."

A nose, alone, is not expressive. It will not seem to suggest or imply a thing about its owner. Alas, a nose must sit in the center of one's face and do battle against a whole set of ideal proportions that are rarely found on real faces. Here are a few that I've come across in various writings on beauty:

The nose should be the same length as the ear.

The nose should tilt slightly upward.

The widest point of the nostrils should be no longer than the distance between the brows.

The classic requirements can seem depressingly endless, but the real trouble lies with our inability to see that these ideal proportions mean nothing on their own. What matters is that the nose works in an interesting, graceful, and eloquent fashion with the rest of the face. When the nose does that the word *classic* becomes unnecessary, leaving room for *flattering*.

Making this feature beautiful is a matter of contouring—of balancing—and of drawing together all of the features to create a look that works. Classic requirements serve us well as guidelines, but the true guide should be the expressive image reflected in a mirror.

LONG NOSE

Seems to pull the face down and elongates space between the eyes and mouth.

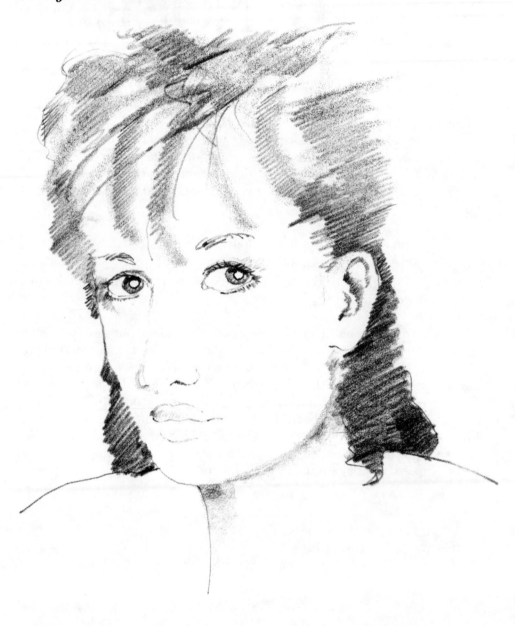

Goal: Through the use of highlighting to focus attention upwards, the nose will seem to assume a shortened, trim shape.

Step 1.   Blend in a touch of highlighter on the bridge between the eyebrows. This will immediately draw attention upwards.

Step 2.   Using the taupe cream, blush rouge or taupe powder, shade the tip of the nose and the sides of the nostrils. This will neutralize the bottom tip, and thus shorten the length of the nose. Shadow carefully, however, and blend into your natural color. Otherwise it will look as though you have a dirty nose!

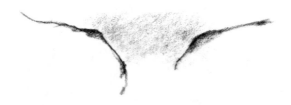

CROOKED NOSE

The sides of the nose are contoured with uneven lines.

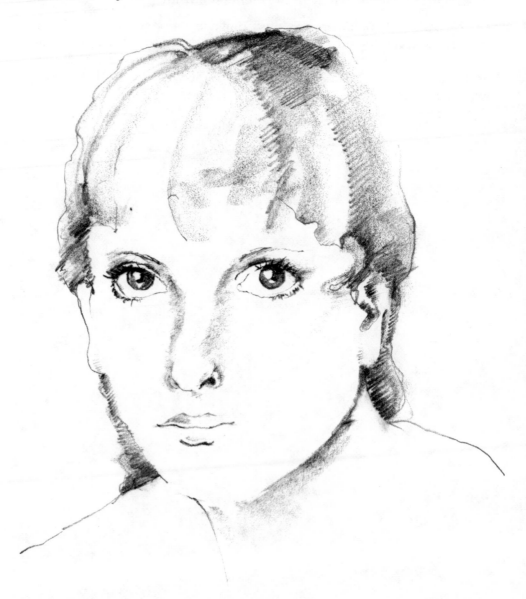

Goal: By using light to bring a curve "out," and shadow to move another "in," the nose will seem more streamlined.

Step 1. Assess the bone structure of your nose as carefully as you can, using your eyes and fingertips to determine the placement of the contours you would like to fix.

Step 2. Highlight the side of the nose you want to move outward, making sure to apply the tone in a clean, neatly blended line. Do not shade onto the cheek.

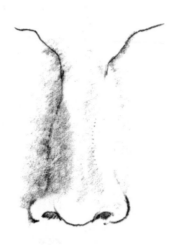

Step 3. On the side of the protruding bulge or bump, apply a taupe shadow and blend onto the nose as far as is necessary to straighten out the line. To achieve a straight line you may have to begin at the inside of the eye socket and move down onto the nostrils.

Common Error: Don't forget the importance of a clean middle line. Because of the complicated shading on either side of the nose, often the line down the center is ignored. The crooked nose will appear to straighten out if there is a clean delineation in the middle.

FLAT NOSE

The sides of the nose seem undefined, the bridge, nonexistent. The contours appear to move out onto the cheeks.

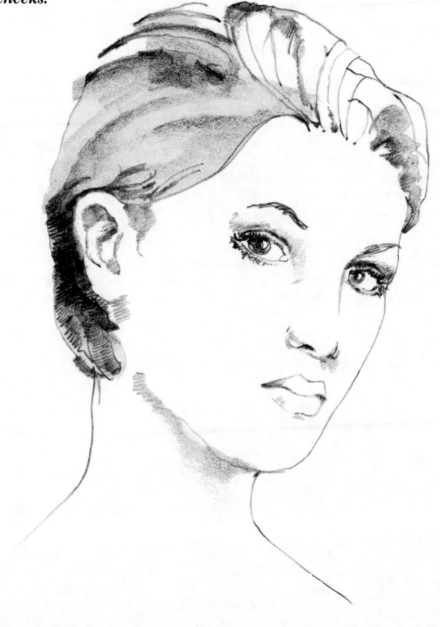

Goal: By using dark and light shadow to sculpt dimension, the nose will take on a more delicate, neatly defined, slimmer shape.

Step 1. Starting from the eye socket if necessary (it will depend on where you perceive the slimming straight contour should begin on your nose) blend a taupe powder or cream cleanly along the sides. Follow the tone gently over the portion of the nostrils that is in keeping with the line. The unstructured sides of the nose will begin to move in.

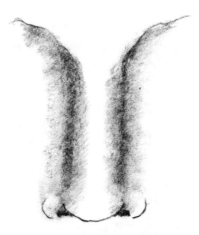

Step 2. Apply a highlighter along the bridge and down the center of the nose, bringing the flat area out. Blend gently into your natural skin tone.

Classic Error: Blend *carefully*. In effect you will have three tones; the taupe or deeper shadow, your own skin tone, and the highlighter. As the dark builds smoothly to the light, the nose will seem to emerge with a more refined shape. If the colors don't build together "naturally," the nose will still appear wide—and striped.

DROOPING TIP

The end of the nose turns down, seeming to pull the other features along with it.

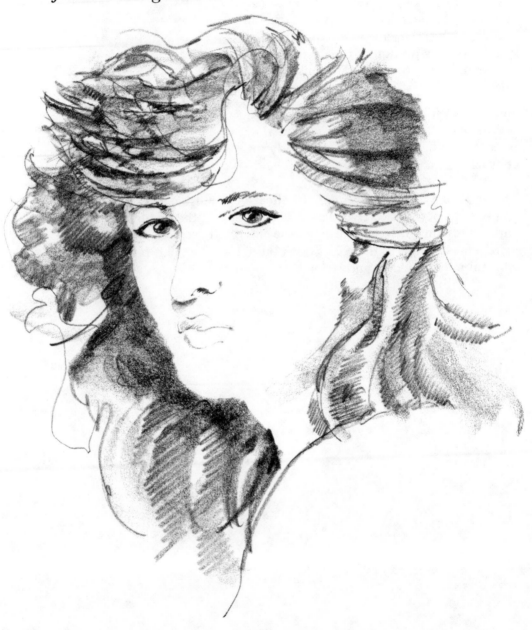

Goal: By applying a deeper tone on and under the drooping contour, the nose will appear to lift up.

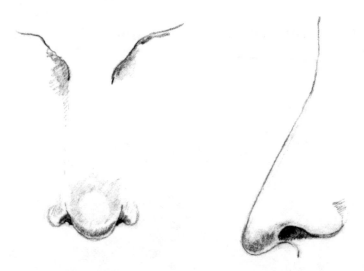

Step 1. Using taupe powder or cream, color the very tip of the nose and under the fold. Do not come up over the tip.

Step 2. Blend in a highlighter, or light base, just over the tip, gently stroking it over the sides. The nose will seem to lift, and the drooping tip will disappear.

WIDE NOSE

The contours seem undefined, and appear to cover a large surface.

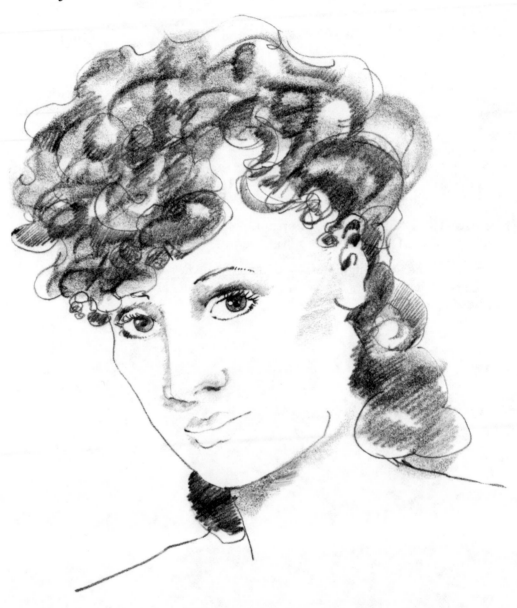

Goal: Contouring shadows will seem to trim the nose, moving the sides in for a slimmer look and a more pleasing, defined line. This requires only one step. With the cream taupe shadow begin at the eyebrow, blend in down through the inner corner of the eye socket, along the side of the nose, and over the nostrils.

Classic Error: Sloppiness. It is crucially important to keep the contouring shadow lines straight. When blending the tones together be sure to do so evenly.

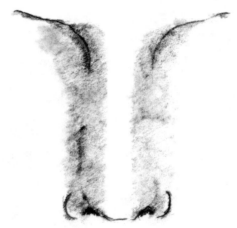

BULBOUS NOSE

Has a large, rounded, often undefined tip.

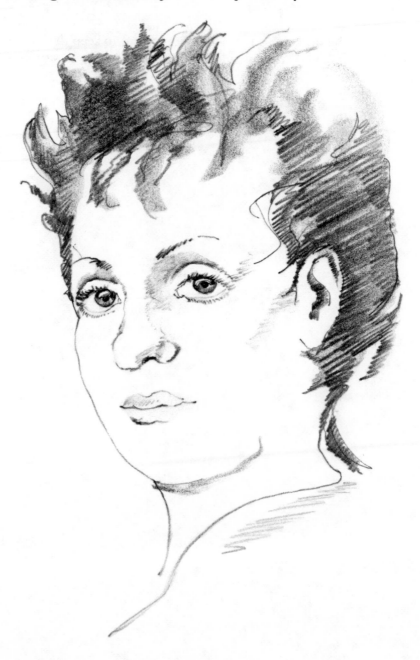

Goal: By using shadow as a delicate sculpting tool, the end of the nose will seem to take on a more angular, defined aspect. The area that appears to sit heavily upon the face, will have a more refined structure.

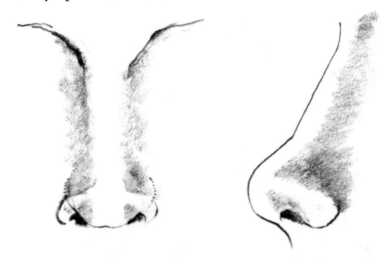

Step 1. Shadow down the sides of the nose with your taupe cream, using a brush and keeping the tone off of the nostrils and away from the eye socket. Bring the shadow to a point, cutting off the sides of the nostrils. Smooth down the sides of the nose, but not out to the cheek.

Step 2. Using the same cream and brush, lightly extend the nostrils to give the effect of a point.

Step 3. Apply a little highlighter down the center of the nose to bring it out. With the darkened sides and the clean, brightened line in the middle, the entire nose from top to bottom will seem more balanced and handsomely sculpted.

Common Error: The kind of contouring that is suggested above works effectively with dim lighting. In bright afternoon or well-lit offices the detailed shadowing may be too obvious. Instead of creating the kind of delicate lines illustrated here, I suggest simply shadowing with the taupe tone down the sides of your nose, applying the color lightly over the sides of the nostrils. Again, highlight cleanly down the center.

PUG NOSE

The tip is clearly turned up.

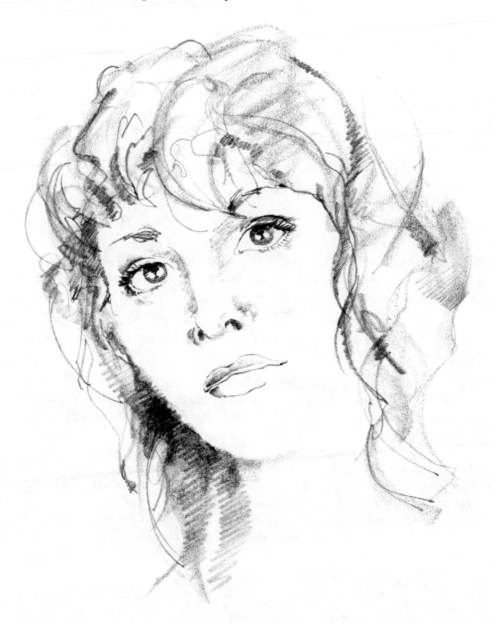

Goal: By tricking the eye with the receding effect of deeper tones, combined with the opening effect of highlighting, the upturned shape of the nose will seem far less obvious.

Step 1. Apply taupe to the tip of the nose and blend down the sides of the nostrils.

Step 2. Place a dot of highlighter right below the shadow on or toward the fold at the bottom of the nose. The upturned portion of the nose, now warmly toned, will seem to move closer to the nostrils, appearing level and smooth.

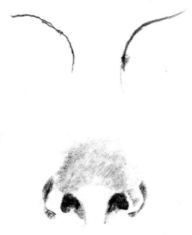

SKI-JUMP NOSE

Seems to move downward in the shape of a slide.

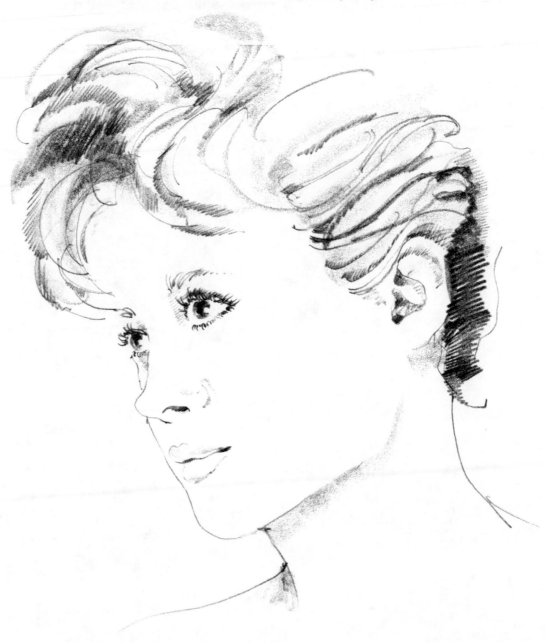

Goal: The sloping outward effect will be minimized as deeper tones bring the nose in, giving it a wider base, and a finite, softly defined tip.

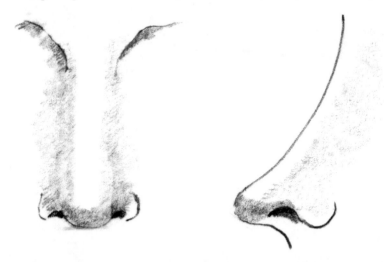

Step 1. Run a line of highlighter down the bridge of the nose, being careful not to sway the tone off on the sides. Feather out very lightly.

Step 2. Using taupe powder, blush, or taupe cream, soften the tip of the nose by bringing the color over and under to the fold. Do not cover the nostrils, but rather gently blend into them, thus bringing the sharper tip in, and the bridge out.

7
FOREHEADS AND JAWLINES

The forehead is a seemingly uncomplicated feature. Yet it is amazing how much it influences the critical balance of the face. It can contribute to an image of delightful harmony or create an uncomfortable imbalance.

Within your makeup routine, then, the forehead is as important as the eyes or lips, and the results of learning to make it up properly can be just as dramatic. Although it seems to be a simple plane, it's a highly malleable feature. Shadow can give it new structure; your hairstyle can also be used as a camouflaging or sculpting tool.

If the face is composed of a series of integrated planes moving in a delicate partnership together to create beauty and interest, then these planes must be defined with a smoothly and gracefully etched line. The chin and jawline—the contours which define the lower portion of the face—are an important part of this line. Again, the issue is balance, but the variations in contour can also effect a "look." *Softness, strength, determination,* and *fragility* are a few of the words that these most expressive contours bring to mind.

The artful use of light and shadow will help you define both this line, and yourself.

HAIR

Hair has often been referred to as a woman's *crowning glory*. It's a poetic notion, yet there is good reason for the term. Hair has the ability to add a flattering touch, to help finish a desired look. But hair also has another capacity. It can effect *change*.

The contours of the forehead, jawline, and cheeks can appear to take on new shape and size with an artful sweep of hair. A very high forehead will quietly disappear, a broad jaw will soften into a gentle oval, and a shapeless cheek will take on new definition. A subtle shift in the hair's length or style can have a powerful sculptural effect on the contours of the face, minimizing the weaknesses and creating new strengths.

Hair is such a valuable *tool* in facial contouring that we might easily have mentioned it earlier in Part I. But hair is also a lovely *feature* that demands the same care and attention as any other. Thus we present it here as both tool *and* feature. A magnificent head of hair is something to be admired and used. Treat it well, and your healthy hair will forever be able to help you *change* your worst feature, and bring out your best one.

LOW FOREHEAD
AND SQUARE JAW

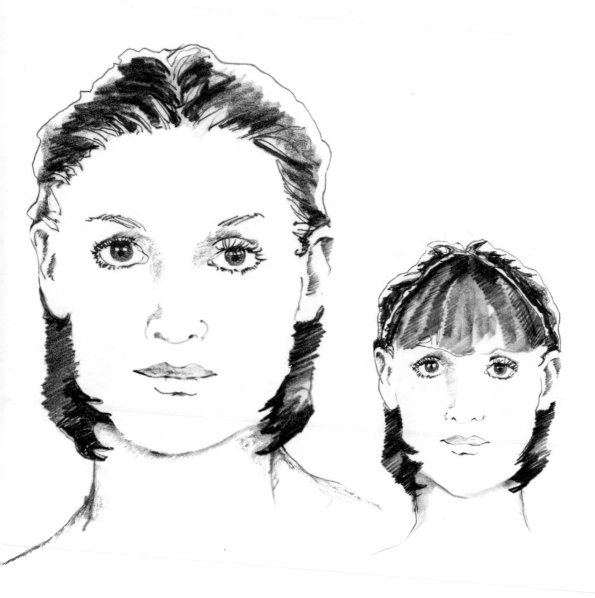

Hair

Keeping hair up and back away from the forehead is one solution. Bangs will also do the job nicely, but they must be cut deep so that the long drop gives the illusion of height. If you would like to have a style that cuts off a piece of the forehead, be sure that there is some lift to the cut around the face; otherwise everything will seem to close in.

Any style that allows the hair to round off the corners of the jaw will be fine. Long or shorter cuts that are styled so that the hair's curl or curve covers the wide edges will give the face the illusion of a lovely oval. If you prefer to wear your hair behind your ears, simply design it so that the hair which tucks behind the ear comes around over the sides of the jaw.

Classic Error: Do not attempt to cover a low forehead with wispy bangs that begin at the hairline. This will only point out the problem.

Makeup

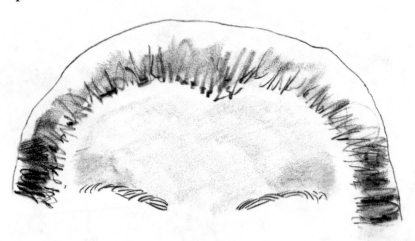

FOREHEAD: Apply highlighter, blending up into the hairline, to create the illusion of an extended space. For a little more dimension, brush on rouge near the temples and above the eyebrows. The three tones, the highlighter, blush, and your natural color, will give you maximum width and will open the forehead right up.

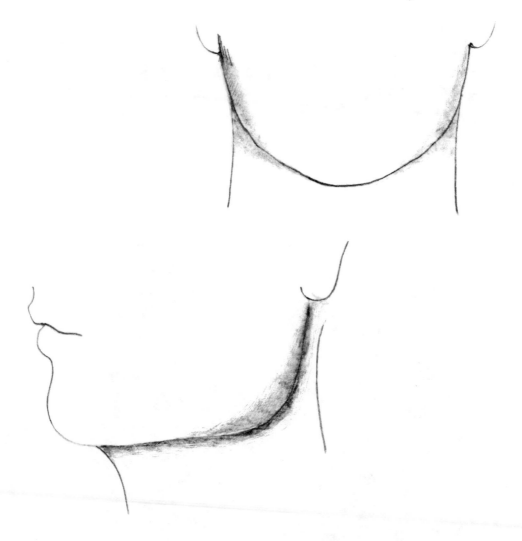

JAWLINE: With a contour powder, color from under the earlobe, up and over the jaw, and underneath the chin. Continue the color lightly around the contours of the square jaw and lightly apply to the neck to camouflage the definition of the edges. Otherwise the shadow should be kept away from the neck. Feather the tone out so that the contouring appears natural and can do the job of softening the sharp lines.

NARROW FOREHEAD AND JUTTING-OUT JAW

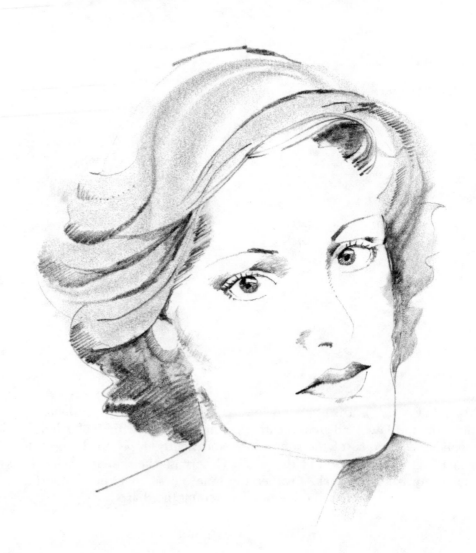

Hair

To create the illusion of a wider forehead, the hair should be swept out at least on one side. By placing an emphasis off-center and away, the eye will be drawn horizontally and out; the forehead will broaden.

Hair can be used easily to detract from a jutting-out jaw by simply drawing attention away from the troublesome contour. The styles that work best are those that are fuller and wider around the eyes and temple, and narrow or closer around the jawline. The look will draw attention upwards, giving the jaw less prominence and minimizing the imbalance.

Classic Error: Do not pull the hair back in an effort to make the forehead seem more expansive. If it's very narrow, it will look very narrow.

Glamour Tip: Highlighting the hair along the temple area with streaks or a lighter color will open out the forehead and give a lovely, sparkling quality to your look.

Makeup

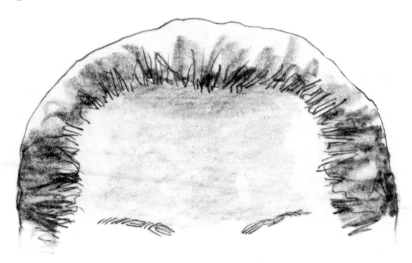

FOREHEAD: To square out, or widen, apply rouge at the hairline (the widow's peak area) in the shape of a half-crescent. Blend in some highlighter at the temples and down the side hairlines. Your natural skin tone in the center (whether or not you apply a base) will seem to move forward and out, creating the illusion of a broader expanse.

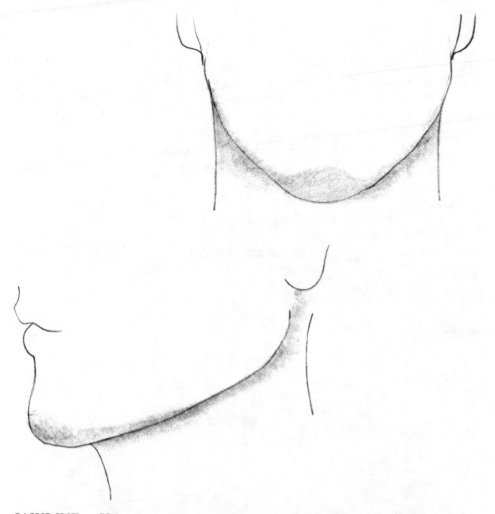

JAWLINE: Using a contour cream or powder, apply color down, under the jaw, and up and over the tip of the chin, so that the jutting-out surface, now less defined, recedes back.

Then, using a blush or taupe cream or shadow, lightly blend the colors back from the chin up to the earlobe. When all of the tones are blended smoothly together, the entire jawline will seem to easily and naturally move back. The face will take on a softer balance.

WIDE FOREHEAD AND POINTED JAW

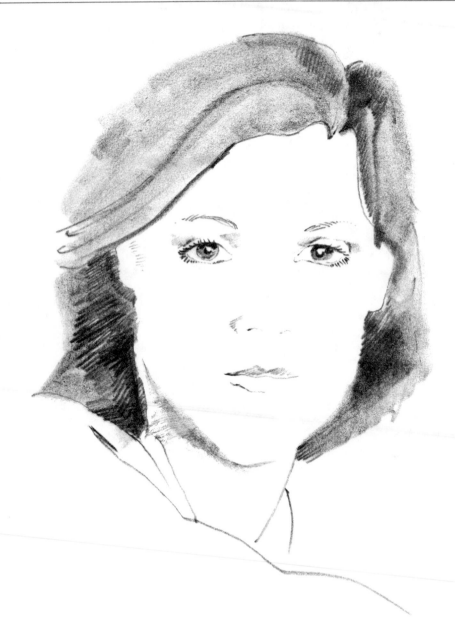

Hair

On a wide forehead hair should be styled to soften the horizontal line and to break off either one or both sides. A side part or a center part will narrow the shape, as long as the line is not a broadly swept one (see "Narrow Forehead"). The hair should be fashioned for a slimming effect.

To flatten out a pointed chin, hair should be kept wide and away from the sharp contour. A cut that is square at the bottom and level with or below the chin will work nicely. Stay away from the shorter cuts; the sloping lines will simply point out the point!

Makeup

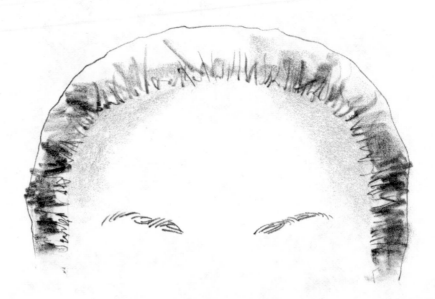

FOREHEAD: Brush half-crescent shapes of rouge or taupe shadow onto the temples, extending the color on either side a third of the way along the hairline of the forehead. Enclosing it all the way is not necessary, as a wide forehead may not necessarily be high. Blend the shadow gently along the edges into your base or natural skin color.

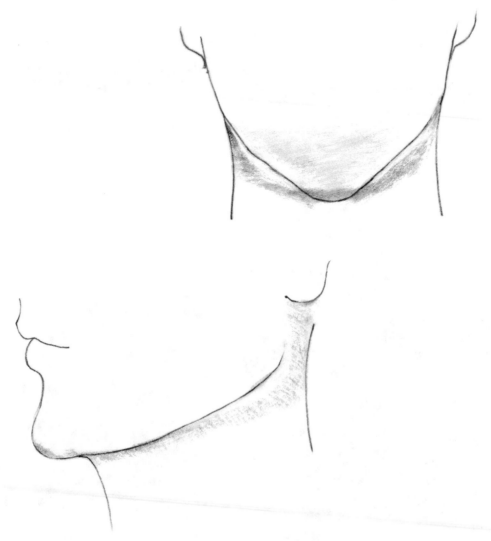

JAWLINE: To square out the point, it may be necessary to "cheat" a little. Using a contour shadow, blend the color straight down from under the ear onto the neck, and follow a line around, up, and over the top of the point. The shape you create need not follow the natural contours of the bone exactly.

Take a light touch of highlighter, and over the corners of the jaw, lighten the areas, blending the color back slightly (not to the jaw hinge!) to flatten and broaden the line.

HIGH FOREHEAD
AND RECEDING JAW

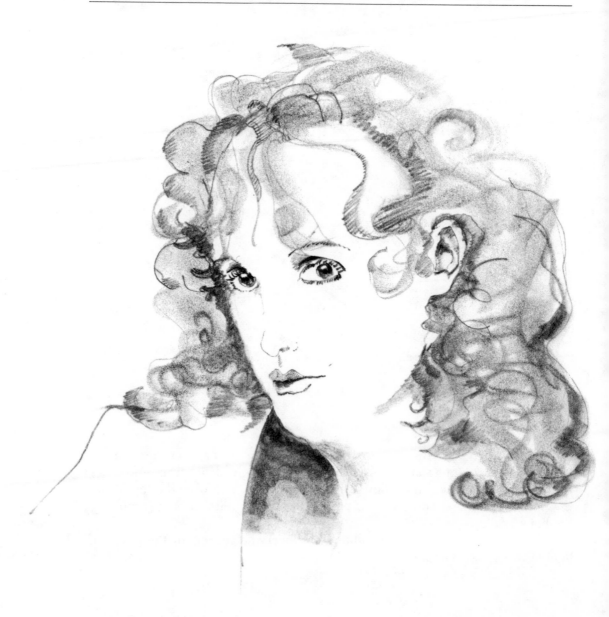

Hair

Perhaps one of the best camouflages for a high forehead is bangs. And your options are many. Bangs needn't be straight china-doll fringes in order to hide the problem. Light, feathered bangs, loose tendrils, or a few wisps may be just enough to break up the expanse.

For a receding chin, the object is to keep the hair from imitating the weak line of the jaw, thereby drawing attention to it. Keep the hair close to the neck, brushed behind or around the ears, and then forward. It can be shoulder length or curve into the middle of the neck. A longer pageboy can work nicely. A hairstyle that offers the face a new contour by either creating a new line, or by hugging the neck rather than the jawline, will do the trick.

Classic Error: Do not forget to study your profile! A high forehead often slopes back. Bangs that cling to this contour no matter how thick or wispy will only worsen the problem. You may need to put a little "lift" in your bangs to give the contour a new dimension.

Makeup

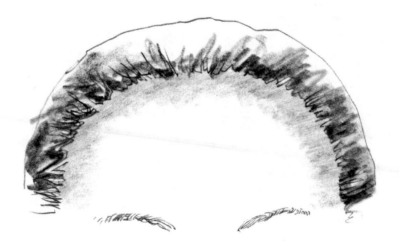

FOREHEAD: Especially if you would like to wear your hair pulled back, apply a contouring shadow or cream into the hairline and blend it lightly toward the center with a brush of rouge. A heavy dome, or simple wide expanse, will seem to disappear.

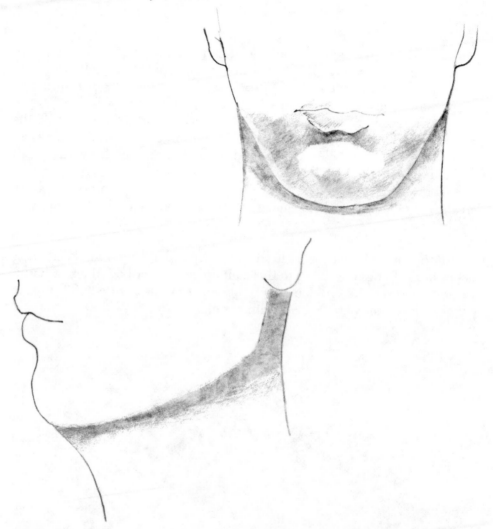

JAWLINE: Starting directly under the earlobe, blend a contouring cream or shadow down onto the neck, and continue the color around underneath the curve of the bone to directly under the chin. Blend the tone underneath the chin onto the neck with a taupe powder or rouge.

Using a highlighter, blend the color into a semicircle on the upper portion of the chin. This light tone next to your natural skin color, juxtaposed to the darker color now under your chin and on the neck, will create a more defined contour.

Apply a little taupe shadow directly under the lower lip for added dimension and strength.

8
NECKS

The neck can be an absolutely majestic feature. The curve of the line, the length, and the grace with which it connects the outer contours of the face to the slope of the shoulders rarely goes unnoticed. This is particularly true for the extremes. The magnificently "swanlike" neck, for example, is unmistakable.

Unfortunately, however, while the neck does not escape a viewer's eye, it frequently remains neglected by its owner. This can be an unflattering mistake. The routines of makeup application should always include attention to the neck. A hairstyle should also be selected with the dimensions of this feature in mind.

It is, after all, a kind of pedestal. If it isn't treated well, the neck will not reflect positively on the face and features it sets off above!

TOO SHORT NECK

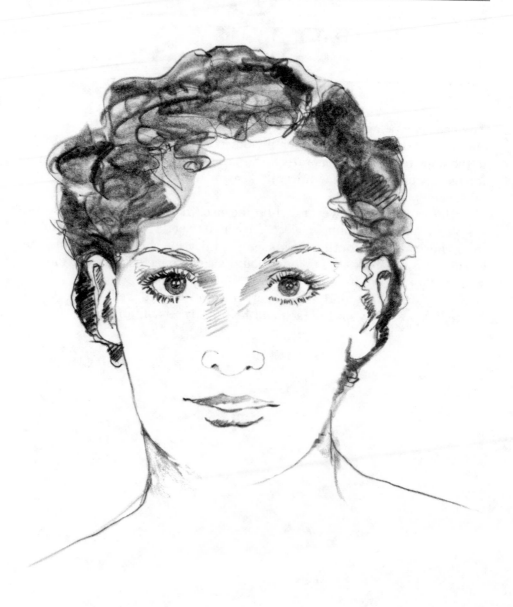

Hair

The hair should be worn up and off the neck. Anything connecting the space between the ears and the shoulders will simply emphasize the short distance between the two.

Makeup

Using a blush, contour shadow, or dark base, lightly color the sides of the neck in the upper corners. This will seem to narrow the top, creating the illusion of a longer line.

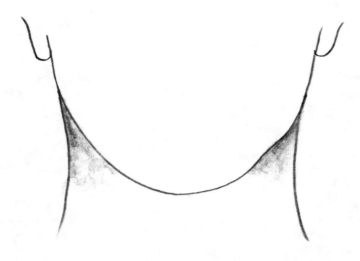

TOO WIDE NECK

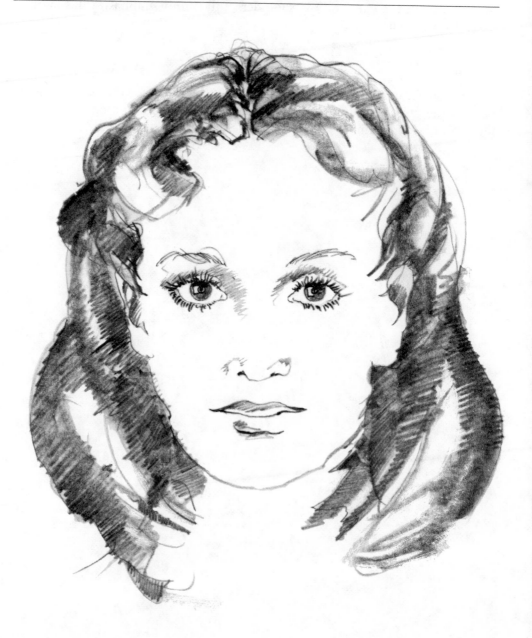

Hair

It's important to choose a style which "cuts" into the neck. Simply selecting long hair to hide the thickness of the neck won't work. Invariably, as you move, it will move too, exposing what you wanted to hide. It may even frame it! But a style which is designed to come in on the neck will move in that direction, covering a measure of the neck's width.

Makeup

Using a blush, contouring shadow, or dark base, shade the side of the neck and bring it up and behind the ear. Blend in.

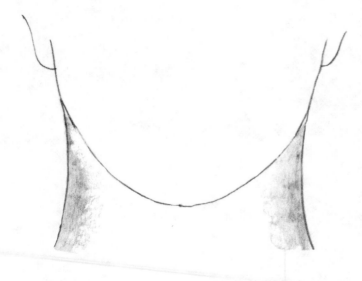

TOO LONG NECK

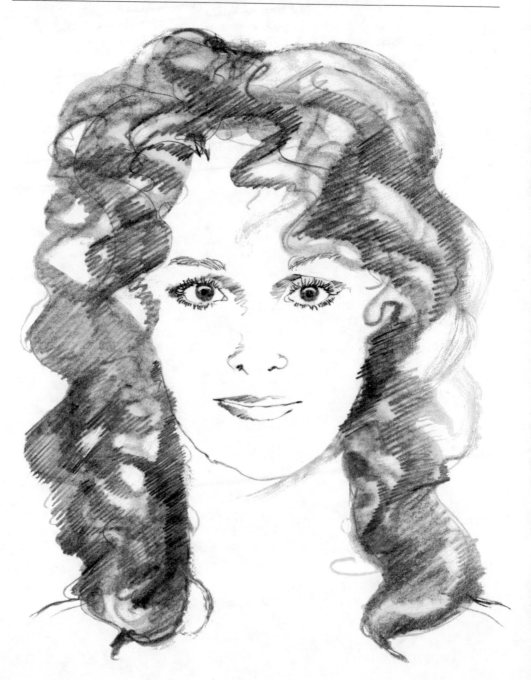

Hair

The hair should be used to close the distance between the ears and shoulders. Longer hair, at least shoulder length, is the best idea, and it should be worn with some width around the neck. If the cut is too slim as it falls below the ears, the neck will only seem longer. The object, of course, is to widen the neck while making it seem less striking in length.

Makeup

Apply a blush, contour shadow, or deep foundation along the top of the neck where the outline of the dip of the chin is most evident. The neck will seem to close in on itself just a little bit.

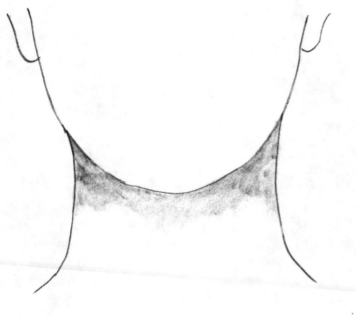

TOO BONY NECK

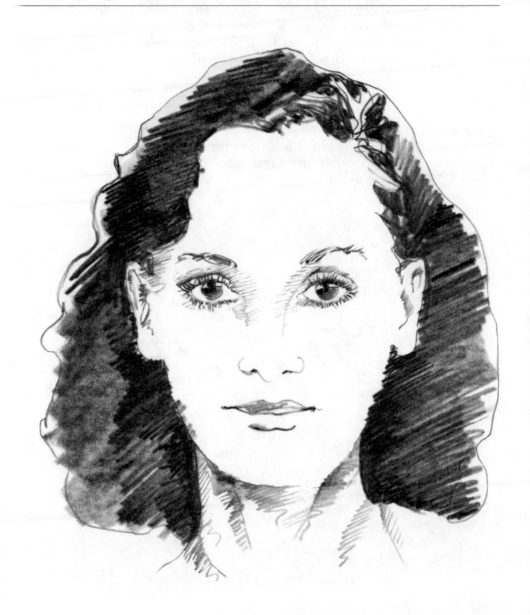

Hair

Styling your hair so that it falls with a nice width at the nape of the neck will draw attention away from the crevices and out to the sides. Attempting to cover the neck may, again, only accentuate the problem. Once you start moving, the hair will fall freely, and the wispy strands which are inevitably left in place might only attract the eye.

Makeup

Along the sides of the neck and up behind the ears, stroke on a base in a color which is lighter than your natural skin tone. It will lend the neck a more solid and substantial look. Then in the two hollows at the front of the neck (a common characteristic of bony necks), lightly apply the base with either your fingertips or a sponge down the center. Blend evenly.

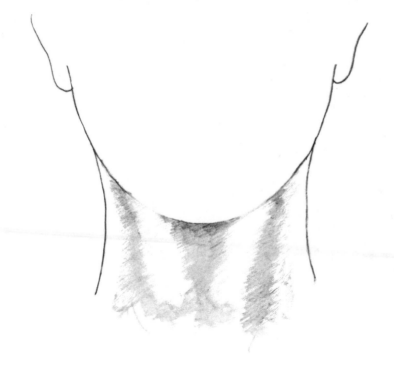

9
CHEEKS

When one thinks of features on the face, the eyes, ears, lips, and nose most frequently come to mind. But there is another feature that has perhaps greater significance or impact, for it has the power to influence the appearance of the parts. It is the *facial contouring*.

The planes of the face, and the interplay of light and shadow they create, lend dimension, balance, delicacy, strength, and interest. When they aren't sharply enough defined or when the contours of the cheek work against the rest of the face, facial contouring can take over. Light and shadow artfully applied to create an illusion of refined and pleasing structure can easily turn an attractive face into an elegant one.

Perhaps more than any other feature, prominent *cheekbones* are the asset every woman wishes to possess. While no one feature on its own can invest a face with refined allure, most viewers will agree that the effect of this graceful contour is striking.

And the good news is, everyone has them. If they are already clear on your face, you may want to bring them forward even more. If they seem absent, subtly drawing them to everyone's attention could help create the look you've always wanted.

HOW TO LOCATE YOUR CHEEKBONES

Place your middle finger on your "sideburn" and slowly follow the bone downward in a diagonal line. Your contouring makeup must be applied in accordance with this, your own bone structure. It's certainly there, you are just going to make it visible! NOTE: sucking in your cheeks does not work. The "line" it creates is invariably too low.

The Most Classic Error: Don't use rouge or blush to actually contour your cheeks. It should be used for color or accent only. Bringing your cheekbones out calls for subtle blending and carefully graduated color. Rouge is anything but that!

TOO FULL CHEEKS

Cheeks seem too rounded, lack angular structure.

Goal: Through the use of contouring shadows and natural rouge tones, the cheeks will take on a more flattering and defined shape and a natural healthful glow.

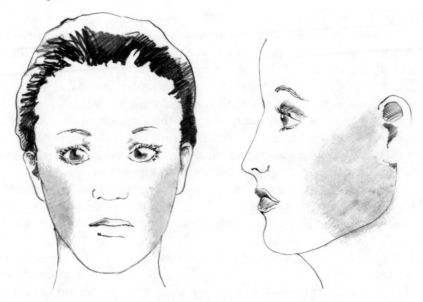

Step 1. Using a deep base (a few shades darker than your natural tone), blend the color down lightly onto the neck and behind the ears.

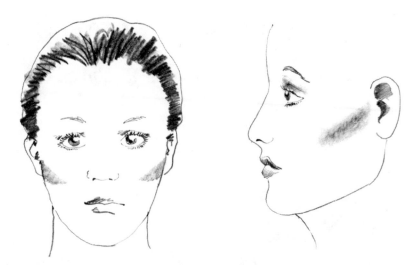

Step 2. Starting at the sideburn and moving directly under the cheek-bone, apply taupe contouring cream or powder. Blend the color down underneath the bone into the darker base. If there is too much clear definition between these tones, blend the contouring color slightly upward. (If you use a cream, remember to powder over it lightly to take away the shine.)

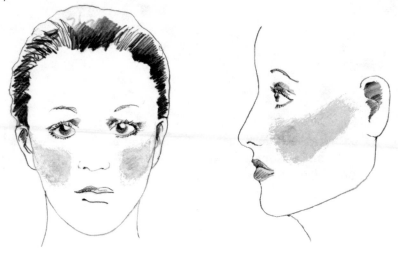

Step 3. Grin. Round shapes will appear. Stroke on your blusher, and then relax the face. With your brush, blend the color upwards above the contouring but slightly over the bone. Leave the space under the eyes as clean as possible.

SHAPELESS CHEEKS

The cheeks seem to have no particular definition.

NOTE:
Almost everything that applies to full cheeks works for this problem.

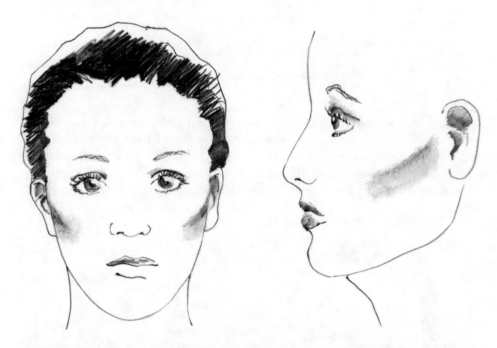

Step 1. Take your middle finger and push down hard at the sideburns. You *will* find a bone. Using a brush-on powder contour, trace a light line just under the diagonal bone you have discovered. To make the line of contour appear natural, blend upward as well as down.

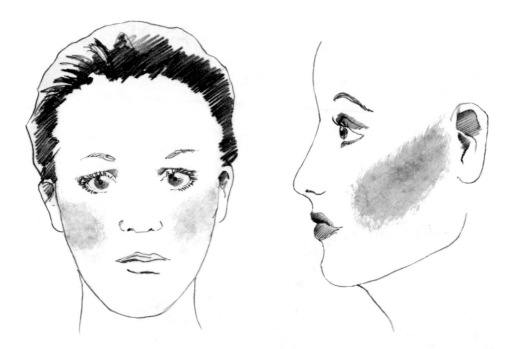

Step 2. Taking your rouge or blush, apply the color to the front of the face, *not* to the sides. Stroke the color close to your nose and up toward the eyes, and above and gently into the contour. Blend the blush into the hairline!

Classic Error: The blush tone you choose should be intense enough to be applied lightly, *not* so light that it must be applied heavily. The faddish style of blushing in bold, heavy streaks looks just like what it is, bold streaks of color. Blush that is gently applied where the cheeks themselves would redden on a brisk day will give you a healthy and natural look. The color should always look as if it is coming from *under* the skin, *not* on top of it.

Glamour Tip: Large button earrings will often seem to make the cheekbones appear more prominent.

SUNKEN-IN CHEEKS

Cheeks seem hollow or concave.

Goal: Here you'll use highlighter to bring the cheeks forward, creating a flatter plane. The rouge, touching up the very front of the cheeks, will also draw attention forward and away from the concave contours.

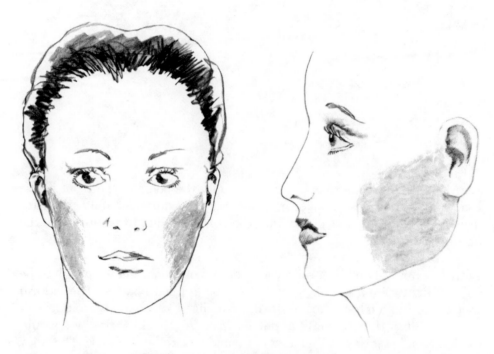

Step 1. Using a highlighter that is slightly lighter in tone than your natural skin tone (but *not* white!), fill in the recessed area, stroking the color back to the ear, down to the jaw, and slightly onto the neck.

114

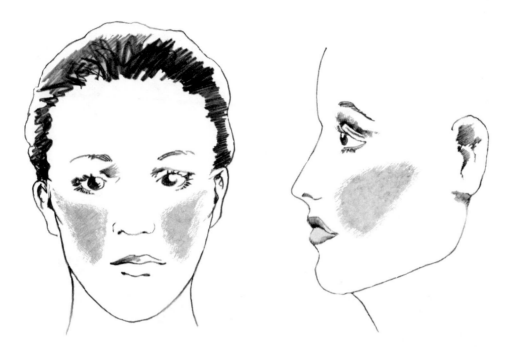

Step 2. Rouge or blush should be concentrated in the front, toward the nose, and down a little toward the jaw. Keep the color *over* the cheekbone.

Classic Error: Do not brush the rouge toward the hairline. It will simply accentuate an already accentuated line.

10
LIPS

There are, of course, the classic lips. The kissable lips, full, but not too full, slightly puckered but not too teasing, richly colored but never "painted." Finally, there are the defined lips—ones that make a graceful statement upon the face by tracing a line of delicate curves and points.

Not everyone's mouth possesses this sort of comeliness. Perhaps this is just as well. Left to their uniqueness, lips are often at their most eloquent. Tempting and suggestive, even when resting motionless, they can truly seem to "speak."

So while the basic idea is to work toward a mouth of graceful, balanced, tempting lines, it is a mistake to ignore completely or try to hide the natural contours of the lips. Your own lips may say far more for you if they are enhanced with light reshaping and warm natural shading than they would painted to resemble a feature that has nothing to do with your own.

Goal: The edges of the mouth are quite precise and therefore difficult to hide. The objective is to give them new definition. Through the use of highlighting, shadowing, and camouflaging, the troublesome natural contours will be deemphasized, while the natural shape of the mouth is preserved. Only then will the lips appear to be naturally yours.

BIG OR FULL LIPS

Seem to overwhelm the other features. Ungraceful in appearance.

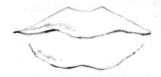 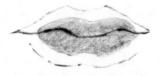

Step 1. Minimize the effect of the full dimensions by covering the entire mouth with a skin-tone press powder or base.

Step 2. To bring attention inside, apply lip gloss or lipstick, fading it outward so that the concentration of color is on the inside of the mouth.

THIN LIPS

Seem to lack shape, contoured with lines more than curves.

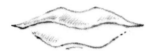 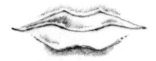

Step 1. Just above the upper lip, following the natural contour, apply a thin pencil line of highlighter in a light pink, almost white color. The lip will seem fuller and more pronounced.

Step 2. Directly under the lower lip apply a line of taupe shadow or pencil to create a more substantial contour. Smudge gently.

Step 3. Use color generously with a lipstick and brush or pencil, following the curves of the lips out to the edges for a voluptuous, richer look.

SMALL LIPS

Seem pursed or tense.

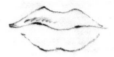 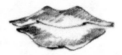

Step 1. Using a lipstick and brush or lip pencil, carry the color out to the extreme corners of the mouth, intensifying the tone on the outside edges.

Step 2. With a base, or lighter color, highlight the center of the upper and lower lip, blending in with your fingers. The darker areas will seem to move outward, creating the illusion of a bigger, more dramatically defined mouth.

Classic Error: Be sure not to extend the color past the lips' natural lines. When the mouth is still it may look fine, but when you begin to speak or smile, it will seem as if the color is "running."

WIDE LIPS

Seem to wander off to the sides and extend onto cheeks.

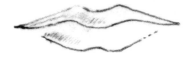 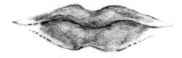

Step 1. Soften the left and right edges of the lips with a skin-tone base or pressed powder.

Step 2. Using a lipstick or gloss applied with a brush, concentrate the color in the center, keeping it away from the outside left and right edges. After creating the shape you want on the inside of the lips, fade the color out at the edges so that the natural wider contours do not work against the new delicate dimensions.

TURNED-DOWN LIPS

The corners of the mouth curve downward.

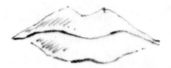 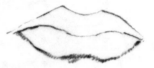

Step 1. Apply the skin tone base or pressed powder to the outside corners to fade the downward curve of the upper lip.

Step 2. Using a light brown or taupe shadow or pencil underneath, follow the lower outside edge, filling in the spaces where the top lip seems to hang over the bottom. Blend the right and left corners carefully so that the lines appear to meet.

Step 3. Using a lipstick and brush, fill in the lower lip completely. Apply the color to the upper lip, keeping away from the outer corners.

UNEVEN LIPS

The lines and curves on the right and left sides are not matched.

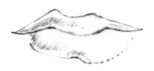 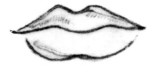 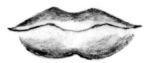

Step 1. Assess your lips carefully, and choose the curve which you prefer and to which you will want to match the other curve. Using a lipstick pencil, trace a contour that complements the "good" side and fill in the lip with lipstick and a brush. Blot the upper lip to blend the colors.

Step 2. Using a taupe shadow or sienna pencil, underline the lower lip, again balancing the side which is the most troublesome to you, and blot. Fill in the lip with lipstick or lip gloss and blend.

A NATURAL-
LOOKING SOLUTION

If you don't like to wear lipstick, you can still correct problem lips. Pat pressed powder over the entire lip area. Then use a damp Q-tip to remove the powder in the shape of a graceful lip outline. Fill in this center area which you have just dabbed free of the powder with a natural lip gloss. Your lips will appear to begin and end exactly where you would like them to.

Classic Errors: Except with the uneven lips, *do not* use a lipstick pencil to harshly draw a new lip contour. Since the edges of the lips are so well defined, the only person you'll be fooling is yourself. Also, *do not* use a lipstick pencil on the outside edge of your upper lip unless the area is free of facial hair. The color will inevitably smudge and will end up creating an uneven and unattractive line. When applying color of any kind to your lips, *do not* start from the center and then move to the sides. Begin at the right and left sides and work inward. This way you will achieve a more balanced line.

Glamour Tip: For a lush and sensuous pair of lips, dot a spot of base on the lower lip and blend. A provocative pout will emerge.

11
EARS

Makeup cannot correct problem ears. This is a feature that either balances well with your face and draws little attention to itself, or overwhelms your facial contours and grabs a bit too much attention.

If your ears work well for you, you could decide to show them. Tuck your hair behind your ears and enjoy! If they don't, you might want to hide them with a flattering hairstyle. And if you can't decide, you can always *disguise* them. Hair can be a useful tool in "reshaping" uneven or large ears. By styling it so that it cuts off a portion of the ears, you will be able to diminish the effects of the offending imbalance.

There is, however, one kind of problem that remains troublesome, despite the options that hairstyles offer: protruding ears. The reason? Either the flaw is *very* dramatic, or the woman simply does not enjoy wearing her hair in a style that masks the problem. Aside from surgery, which, of course, is an option for everyone, *glueing* is probably the best solution.

Step 1. Spirit gum, which is made of resin from tree sap, and can be bought in a theatrical supply store, should be applied to the back inner portion of the ear. Spread the glue all the way back to the line where the ear and skull connect.

Step 2. Hold the ear down for a few minutes with either your hand or by lying on your side. It *will* stay—for days—but it is not advisable to leave the glue on for more than a few hours. The substance can be removed with alcohol.

Common Error: You must remember to test for any allergies. Simply dab a little of the spirit gum to your arm, leave it on for an hour or so, and remove. If there's no reaction within the next few hours, go ahead and flatten those ears!

Conclusion

In *Special Features*, I have tried to relate the important issues, techniques, and goals of beauty as I see them. I have been able to offer information on colors, techniques of application, contouring principles, tips on common errors, and suggestions for glamorous touches. But my advice can go only so far: what counts more than any piece of information I can offer is *your approach*.

I've shown you all the tools you will need to find the hidden beauty in your face. But as I said before, any book on beauty is incomplete, because it must treat in a finite way something that has infinite possibilities. Now you need to experiment, practice, and enjoy—by doing so you will make this book limitless.

The answers are here, but only you can find them and even change them when you seek a new solution to your own beauty problems. I hope that *Special Features* will give you the freedom to see what you can do for yourself and by yourself with ease and pleasure.

Trust what you see. If I were applying your makeup, your vision of yourself would certainly be an important guide. Now it's up to you.